HANDBOOK OF
OSTEOPATHIC TECHNIQUE

HANDBOOK OF
OSTEOPATHIC TECHNIQUE
Second edition

Laurie S. Hartman
DO, MRO
Head of Department of Osteopathic Technique,
British School of Osteopathy, London

HUTCHINSON
London Melbourne Sydney Auckland Johannesburg

Hutchinson & Co. (Publishers) Ltd

An imprint of the Hutchinson Publishing Group

17-21 Conway Street, London W1P 6JD

Hutchinson Publishing Group (Australia) Pty Ltd
16-22 Church Street, Hawthorn, Melbourne, Victoria 3122

Hutchinson Group (NZ) Ltd
32-34 View Road, PO Box 40-086, Glenfield, Auckland 10

Hutchinson Group (SA) (Pty) Ltd
PO Box 337, Bergvlei 2012, South Africa

First published by NMK Publishers 1983

Second edition published by Hutchinson 1985

Printed and bound in Great Britain by
Anchor Brendon Ltd, Tiptree, Essex

British Library Cataloguing in Publication Data

Hartman, Laurie S.
    Handbook of osteopathic technique — 2nd ed.
    1. Osteopathy
    I. Title
    615.5'33   RZ341

ISBN 0 09 160680 2

CONTENTS

A carefully educated sense of touch is the keynote to both osteopathic diagnosis and operative technique. From the very nature of the osteopathic conception, the physical body is viewed as a mechanism whose disordered or diseased conditions demand anatomical readjustment; it is imperative that a delicate and educated sense of touch be acquired in order to apply its tenets logically and successfully.

The Practice of Osteopathy, McConnell and Teal.

PREFACE

This book is aimed at all those engaged in that branch of the healing arts dealing with manual therapy. Although primarily written for students and graduates of osteopathy, it is hoped that it may help to transcend the somewhat artificial barriers that exist between different practitioners of varied disciplines who are using manipulative methods.

I am of the opinion that no particular group has the sole right to perform manipulative procedures. Each discipline of manual therapy has its advantages and its disadvantages due to emphasis in particular directions. It is the purpose of this book to try to show the broad spectrum of techniques used by osteopaths and therefore to further proliferate knowledge and discussion for the ultimate benefit of the patient.

I owe a considerable debt of gratitude to many people without whose help this book would never have reached publication. To name just a few, my thanks are due to Michael Hunt, who is currently a student at the British School of Osteopathy, who so successfully took the photographs using his professional photographic skills. My thanks go also to my daughter Nicola, Katheryn West and Amos Shannan, recent graduates at the B.S.O. who modelled on many Sunday afternoons in their own time for the photographs. Finally, I should like to thank my wife Jennifer, who so laboriously typed the notes repeatedly for this book.

Comments and errata are welcomed.

July 1983
Laurie Hartman
Head of Department of
Osteopathic Technique
British School of Osteopathy
1-4 Suffolk Street
London SW1

How to use this book

It is virtually impossible to learn osteopathic technique or any other form of manual therapy purely from the written word and photographs. However this book is designed to act as an *aide-memoire* and also should be a means of learning the basic holds or positions for application of the hands. The conversion of these into living techniques can be developed with personal tuition at a later stage without the inevitable fumbling and difficulty in trying to remember which usually occurs with any new skill.

Terminology varies according to the discipline of the practitioner and I have attempted to conform to standard anatomical terminology throughout and tried to avoid jargon wherever possible for the sake of clarity. The chapter on the classification of osteopathic technique should assist any problems of language.

It is impossible to show the dynamic aspects of any form of procedure in static photographs. To try to combat this problem some use has been made of sequences of pictures to assist in clarifying difficult points. In several places the hands have been shown separate from their application to further aid clarification.

Most of the photographs have arrows added to them, not to show specific directions, but to show the general direction in which forces are being applied. It should be noted that most of the arrows are curved as in fact in the body there are of course no straight lines and most forces have to be directed along an arc. No importance should be attached to the size of the arrows, they are purely for clarification purposes.

It is suggested that the reader acquaint himself with the classifications of osteopathic techniques and the modifying factors before trying to unravel the finer details of the pictures.

As the current emphasis in teaching at the British School of Osteopathy (B.S.O.) is in the use of as low a force as is possible, combined with as little leverage as will be successful, some of the positions will not appear on first viewing to be effective as technique procedures to achieve the declared objective. However if the reader will try to duplicate the position as accurately as possible on a partner he will find that he is using a series of very efficient and effective techniques which are uniquely non-traumatic.

Not all techniques are suitable for all patients or indeed to be performed by all operators. For a small operator, performing some of the techniques requiring them to take a considerable portion of the patient's weight, is obviously impractical. All techniques can be modified according to the patient, his general state of health, his age, sex, mental state, and the degree of pain he is in at a given time. It is not the function of this book to enter into aspects of diagnosis and actual choice of time for application of particular techniques but purely to aim at cataloguing a range of approaches.

Thrust techniques are potentially dangerous in certain cases and in certain conditions and it is suggested that no attempt be made to use these without the benefit of personal instruction or considerable experience in their use. Osteopaths have an admirable safety record in this regard and this is mainly due to the long painstaking practice they undergo as students spending many hours training in manipulative techniques on each other before they graduate to handling patients.

The spectrum of osteopathic techniques includes a number of "reflex" techniques and no attempt has been made to illustrate these although they are included in the section on classification. This is because it is considered essential to have personal tuition in these methods to make them effective.

The author feels similarly about cranial techniques although there are specialist texts available in that field with the theories and practical approaches.

SOMATIC DYSFUNCTION

The term "Osteopathic lesion" has been largely replaced by the use of the term "Somatic Dysfunction". This seems to have come about due to the realisation of the existence of a palpable entity of mechanical disturbance in the structure of the body by professions other than the osteopathic. There is a problem when referring to either term, which should be fully interchangeable, of defining what exactly is being referred to. A lesion may be primary, or secondary. A primary dysfunction may be due to trauma, either as a single incident or as a result of a series of micro-traumata. However if the repeated micro-traumata are occasioned by the presence of a dysfunction elsewhere in the structure, then we have a situation of secondary dysfunctioning. We then have a primary dysfunction at one point but a similar palpable entity elsewhere which is in fact a secondary lesion, dependent, at least initially on the primary. Thus a secondary lesion in this sense is really an adaptation to some intrinsic fault in the mechanics of the structure. An adaptation which cannot fully compensate will go on to become a compensation, which is in fact dysfunctional, whereas an adaptation is a normal physiological response. It is only unsuccessful adaptive processes which lead to the need for compensation in the musculo-skeletal system in this sense.

What converts an adaptation to a compensation is open to some dispute. Sometimes it is due to patterns "learnt" by muscles, sometimes due to perverted function producing physiological modifications which become pathological. This later entails the alteration of the material properties of the collagenous and elastic connective tissues that make up the tendons, ligaments, fascial and other structures surrounding an articular unit. Some of these changes are not capable of spontaneous resolution once they have passed a certain stage and it is then that manipulative treatment is the important modality over most others. If muscle or fascia is too short due to compensatory mechanisms there will be a tendency for reduced movement in adjacent joints and subsequent dysfunction can develop. If the demands of body mechanics are for flexibility, there will be a tendency for compensatory hypermobility in some areas, with its attendant symptomatology.

The other type of secondary lesioning is that sort due to altered reflex pathways from the presence of perverted viscero-somatic reflexes emanating from a dysfunctional viscus. The nature of the palpable findings in these cases will be somewhat different. The tissues will have a characteristic "doughy" nature and the nature of the palpable joint dysfunction will be more "springy" than those in a purely mechanical case. If however the situation is maintained for long enough there may be adaptive changes in the somatic tissues which do not restore to normal when the primary irritation from the C.N.S. has gone.

Asymmetry is the rule rather than the exception when dealing with the human structure. Nevertheless asymmetry which is dysfunctional is significant as it is often a source of symptoms, if not locally, then possibly at remote sites. We are left therefore with having to define what is relevant in objective findings. Quality of disturbance is seen to have far greater significance than quantity. Imbalance of action around a moving part has to be diagnosed by examining the part in motion. Static examination can only give a part of the picture. The aim of treatment should therefore be to help the patient's structure become more able to adapt itself to the environment. It is assumed in this respect, that a structure which is working harmoniously is more efficient and less likely to be a source of symptoms.

The chief governing factor is that function governs comfort.

1

TREATMENT PRINCIPLES

Osteopathic technique and osteopathic treatment are not synonymous. New techniques are constantly being originated, modified and added to the repertoire. Nevertheless the basic principles underlying the technical approach to osteopathic structural therapy conform to certain basic principles which can be classified and analysed for identification and teaching purposes.

Osteopathic technique can be said to consist of passive movement applied manually to the body for the purpose of adjusting mechanical derangements in anatomical structures found by various examining procedures to be functioning at less than their optimum. The number of techniques is really infinite because the guiding factors are the tissues that the osteopath is working on. However, the broad principles underlying these particular approaches are finite and it is these which govern our classifications of approach. The guidelines of a particular technical procedure are the anatomical limits of motion possible in a particular part being worked on. A large number of techniques have evolved which have a basic procedural outline common to many operators. These procedures can be used as an empirical "manipulation" in which case they tend to be rather hit and miss, but the basic technique, if analysed thoroughly, will be found to be made up of a number of components which can be varied in many subtle ways. The particular skill of the osteopath lies in the ability to adapt these techniques using very accurate palpation sense and sympathetic feel for the tissues, to the patient and the condition that he presents with. This comes from the utilisation of the deployment of modifications made possible by variations in all the components of forces which make up the given procedural technique. Attempts to copy the techniques in outline without understanding the principles will only meet with limited success as the modifications adapt the technique not only to the palpatory findings, but the diagnostic features as a whole, thus making provision for restrictions and contra-indications imposed by the patient's physique, age, temperament and any local or general degenerative or pathological changes.

In fact there is no such thing as osteopathic technique. Manipulative methods regardless of the discipline of the practitioner are totally guided by the raw material we have to work with, i.e. the human body. However osteopaths have two major advantages over most of the other groups. These are, firstly, that as a system, osteopathic manipulative methods have been in existence longer than most, if not all of the others. Secondly, we utilise a degree of delicacy in palpation and tissue awareness and "tissue tension" sense that enables us to combine diagnosis, assessment and therefore choice of approach in a somewhat unique way.

Without getting too deeply embroiled as to the hypothesis underlying the need for manipulative treatment, the majority of manipulators, if they are honest with themselves are working primarily on joints within the body that have some limitation of their function, usually also combined with adjacent areas of muscular hypertonus. A broad general rule could be stated, that function governs comfort. The type of loss of function leads to the diagnosis, or assessment in a mechanical sense of the structure or structures involved in a particular dysfunction, and therefore the choice of technique to attempt to restore the functional integrity. A cardinal rule of osteopathy is that structure governs function, and of course the two are totally linked and interdependent. Altered structural mechanics can lead to altered function of an area. This may not at the time be a source of symptoms but can enter into a gross compensation pattern which can be broken down by future superimposed strains etc. Any technique of treatment can only be empirical unless it is based on a diagnosis. Osteopathic diagnosis can be classified as a method of differentiation between a mechanically well adapted human structure which is capable of functioning normally in its environment, and a structure unable to adapt itself to its environmental demands because of internal disease or disorder, poorly compensated body mechanics, or misuse of the structure. These abnormalities can become a cause of symptomatology in themselves or lead to a predisposition to disease or disorder.

Case history taking, particularly emphasising aggravating and alleviating factors in symptomatology, is essential in osteopathic practice. Physical examination of a detailed nature, including a particularly searching palpatory investigation, is also part of the usual osteopathic diagnostic method. The history, observation and examination should enable a determination of which tissue or tissues, in whatever functional or pathological state, are causing the symptoms. The predisposing factors leading up to this particular breakdown should also have been assessed. The type of treatment best suited to the individual can be decided on, and if osteopathic treatment is considered appropriate, the plan of treatment can be made up. The use of as accurate a prognosis as is possible is emphasised to act as confirmation of diagnosis and to give the patient some idea of the outcome of any treatment plan.

Absolute and relative contra-indications to particular techniques must be observed and a trained, thinking practitioner should never take unnecessary risks with his patient's welfare.

Passive movement testing of accessory ranges of joint movement as well as physi-ological ranges is seen as essential, but the main emphasis in palpatory diagnosis should be on accurate tissue tension sense to assess the quality of a particular dysfunction and in this way, although technique can never be totally divorced from diagnosis, it can almost be used as a therapy as one is using pre-technique trial positions as part of the functional analysis.

When planning a treatment as a combination of different techniques applied to a particular tissue or tissues a constant awareness of the diagnosis and the requirements of the tissues at that particular time should be uppermost in the mind. The whole exercise should be an attempt to co-operate with nature as exhibited in a given patient at that time in an effort to restore as much harmonious working to that patient's system as it is capable of. This leads them back to a state of relative ease as good as, if not better than, before they became diseased. Treatment should therefore never be rushed and violent but should be of the gentlest possible variety capable of giving the required result. Adverse reactions to treatment are a warning and should lead to reasessment to discover any possible concealed pathology etc.

CLASSIFICATION OF OSTEOPATHIC TECHNIQUES

Osteopathic techniques fall very broadly into three main categories. These are somewhat arbitrary divisions due to an attempt to try to classify them for teaching purposes. The current system used at the B.S.O. is one of dividing techniques into categories based on the actual application of forces rather than on what is trying to be achieved or on some supposed action.

Rhythmic techniques fall into eight groups.
1. Kneading
2. Stretching
3. Articulation
4. Rhythmic Traction
5. Springing
6. Inhibition
7. Vibration
8. Effleurage

Thrust techniques can be divided into five categories.
1. Combined leverage and thrust.
2. Momentum induced modification of combined leverage and thrust.
3. Minimal leverage modification of combined leverage and thrust.
4. Non leverage thrust.
5. Momentum induced modification of non leverage thrust.

Low velocity stress techniques can be divided into four main categories.
1. Low velocity stress using sustained leverage.
2. Low velocity stress using sustained pressure.
3. Low velocity stress using sustained traction.
4. Low velocity stress using sustained articulation.

A planned approach is encouraged, to try to produce less tendency to random techniques and produce a reproducible result with recordable approaches using named techniques; the aim being to help enable the patient's system to readjust towards a normal compensation for the environment and mechanical needs. Some uniformity in terminology is encouraged to aid recording of treatment methods for inter-operator consistency of approach and dialogue.

The need for postural advice, exercises for flexibility and muscle strengthening, advice on environment at home, and at work, is of course equally a part of osteopathic management in patient care. Other modalities from experts in fields other than osteopathic technique may of course be needed in certain cases and the trained osteopath is aware of comparative therapeutics. Nevertheless the osteopath has a unique part to play in any treatment team because of his detailed diagnostic methods developed over the years and because of his safe, effective manipulative methods.

Rhythmic Techniques
These can be classified as repetitive procedures where the control of rhythm plays an essential part. The forces are applied and released in a graduated fashion.

1. Kneading
This is usually a slow rhythmical movement combined with pressure; it is applicable to skin, fascia, muscle etc. depending on the speed and the depth of the pressure. The usual rhythm is somewhere around 10–15 cycles per minute. This can be increased to produce a stimulatory, as distinct from a relaxing response up to approximately 36 cycles per minute but rarely any faster. Kneading can be applied superficially or deeply, over a small or a large area and is usually a cross fibre movement. Therefore, a knowledge of the anatomy of the attachments of the tissues being worked is important and the type of handling is critical. Pinching the skin produces adverse reaction and patient resistance and is therefore to be avoided. The most effective type of kneading is that which will produce the maximum relaxation of the muscle being worked on in the shortest possible time and this is usually achieved with a slow, unhurried, deep pressure just short of discomfort, sensed by the operator's hand constantly monitoring the tissue response.

The applicator with which this technique

is applied is most usually the thenar eminence or hypothenar eminence of the operator's hand. Finger-tips or points of thumb are rarely used in this technique as they are uncomfortable for the patient and extremely hard on the operator.

The depth of effect is governed as much by the operator using body weight as it is by the actual force applied by the hand itself. The sense of relaxation of muscle is best palpated by the operator's own joint proprioceptive mechanism rather than by the tactile sensory apparatus in the finger-tips. Each operator will find his own most comfortable rate and pressure as applied to a particular patient, but a very rough average would be approximately 30 pounds pressure when applied to the spinal muscles of a well built man. This would of course have to be modified accordingly with small, light, frail, or very young or nervous patients etc.

2. Stretching
This is once again a slow rhythmic technique employing separation of muscle attachments, stretch of the ligaments, fascia, membrane etc. The tissue reached can be affected by the amplitude of the stretch. For example a short amplitude stretching technique would be aimed at the short intra-articular structures of an individual spinal segment. However a longer amplitude technique would be aimed to stretch extrinisic structures to a particular joint or area of the spine. Of course an intimate knowledge of the anatomy of the attachments of the structure one is working on is important, the type of handling is critical and once again a slow, purposeful, gradually applied increasing force will usually produce the most rapid relaxation and change in the underlying tissues. The rate of application of the forces in stretching techniques is similar to those in kneading techniques. Sometimes a final small extra stretch at the end of each movement is used as this produces a quicker release of tension.

3. Articulation
This very old osteopathic terminology could be classified as repetitive passive movement usually employing the use of a lever and fulcrum to enhance the power without the need for high applications of force. The difference between articulation and simple passive movement is that the operator should be constantly sensing the feed-back from the tissues under his hand and measuring and gauging the intensity of pressure and stretch necessary according to what he is feeling.

Articulation can be performed over a wide arc or over a very small amplitude of movement according to the treatment prescription for the case. Taking a shoulder repeatedly from a few degrees of abduction into full abduction would be an example of a wide range. Taking a particular lumbar segment from almost full flexion to its complete range would be a good example of a small range of articulation. Often articulatory techniques are combined with a small emphasis of movement right at the end. This little "bounce" is a very useful way of producing more rapid change in tissues as well as assessing the reactivity in the tissues as they are moved at different rates.

4. Rhythmic Traction
By this term we mean manually applied repetitive attempts to separate and release joint surfaces and produce stretch of inter- and peri-articular structures. Osteopaths rarely use mechanical aids and rhythmic traction will produce relaxation in tissues very quickly when performed slowly and carefully, preferably with one hand monitoring the part we wish to stretch. It is often performed after thrust techniques and articulatory techniques to utilise the lubricating effect of synovial fluid which occurs after the separation of joint surfaces. This refractory period of relative hypermobility after thrust techniques is very useful as the synovial fluid thins out for a short while and articulatory techniques can gain greater ranges of movement than they could in normal circumstances.

5. Springing
By this term we mean repetitive pressure of a graduated nature applied to a bony landmark and is sometimes combined with very short leverages. Rarely is springing applied quickly, more often a slow rhythmical pressure and release using the proprioceptive mechanism in the applicator and in the operator's arm and body to sense the point at which the release is achieved. Springing is used as a diagnostic technique over spinous processes to assess tenderness, resistance, and reactivity.

6. Inhibition
This is the only term which actually states what we are trying to achieve as distinct from what we are applying to the patient and this is another very old osteopathic term which

we retain by common usage. In practice it consists of pressure applied for fairly long periods being slowly and deeply brought into play and then slowly and gradually released. It is usually applied over a small area, occasionally over bony points, or areas of the body where the inhibitory effect is considered necessary. The rhythm of inhibition is always slow and needs a constant awareness of tissue reaction. It is usually applied with a gradually increasing pressure at the same or similar rate as the patient's respiration. An example of inhibition would be deep pressure applied with the point of the thumb over the inferior attachment of levator scapulae in a case of acute torticollis. As with all other rhythmical techniques a feed-back from the tissues is essential. When considering inhibition, the opposite, i.e. stimulation, comes to mind. Any technique can be made "stimulatory", although it is important to differentiate between stimulation and "irritation". To separate the two is often difficult and for this reason we do not usually include stimulation in our categories of techniques. If there is a specific intention to produce irritation in tissues which are hypotonic and slack, then well and good. However if inhibition is the aim then great care must be taken not to over-stimulate with excess pressure. Inhibition is designed to produce relaxation, improvement in local circulation, and reduction in facilitation of afferent impulse response, so irritation is in fact the opposite of this.

7. Vibration
We include the use of manually applied rapid oscillatory pressure or movement in our techniques. There are sometimes occasions when its use over hollow structures such as nasal sinuses is useful. It is usually applied superficially and at a fairly fast rate.

8. Effleurage
This technique, borrowed from the massage armamentarium, is included in our list of rhythmic techniques, because there are many occasions when a rhythmically applied movement of light force and slow rate are necessary. It is usually used on the superficial tissues to produce a "drainage" effect on lymphatic channels and is thus most commonly applied from peripheral toward central tissues. It is often used over areas where congestion is considerable to produce a circulatory response to aid decongestion and produce counter-irritation. Osteopaths generally do not use lubricants when they perform their techniques but in effleurage some form of skin oil will prevent soreness, aid movement and make the technique easier.

Thrust Techniques
These much maligned techniques can be defined as the rapid application of force, the primary objective being to direct that force along a given plane to a given point, area, or structure. Thrust techniques do not necessarily have to be carried out at the limit of a range of movement. With sufficient speed joint "gapping" can be achieved even in the middle ranges of joint play without any trauma being induced. They are usually applied parallel or at right angles to the plane of the articulation and in a direction against the barrier of joint fixation. This is usually done with varying degrees of leverage to place the joint in the most favourable position. Sudden movement of the joint by thrust or leverage or combinations of both produces the characteristic sound.

There five broad sub-divisions of thrust techniques by our current classification.
1. Combined leverage and thrust.
2. Combined leverage and thrust using momentum.
3. Minimal leverage.
4. Non leverage thrust.
5. Non leverage thrust using momentum.

1. Combined leverage and thrust
In this technique, a thrust is applied at or near the point of lesion, with or without application of exaggeration of leverage at the thrust point. As an alternative a thrust could be applied at or near the extremity of a lever arm remote from the lesion. A static fulcrum may be created by pressure or fixation at or near the lesion.

(a) Thrust at the lesion point. A typical cervical thrust technique employing side-bending with "reverse" rotation with the patient supine, sitting etc.

(b) Thrust at the extremity of a lever arm. An example of this would be a supine mid-dorsal thrust technique where the operator's hand is placed under the patient's body and a thrust is applied to the patient's arms placed in various ways across the chest.

(c) Combination thrust at lesion point and at extremity of lever arm. An example of this variation would be a sitting mid-dorsal, knee in the back technique, this being done with the operator's hands clasped round the patient's wrists where their hands are clasped behind their neck.

2. Momentum induced thrust
This method is really a sub-division of the previous category but using momentum or movement. The operator uses a build-up of momentum in the primary leverage direction several times until he senses that the summation of levers is optimum. It is particularly useful for heavily built patients, and for very rigid areas. The main part of the leverage is applied and released several times in succession and the thrust is applied as the patient is in a relaxed phase or as the movement builds up to a suitable level at the lesion point. This has the advantage that the patient and the operator are gently on the move and the point of optimum tension can be much more readily felt by the operator's own proprioceptive mechanism. It does however have the disadvantage that there can be a tendency to lose control of the amplitude and this can make the technique needlessly powerful and potentially traumatic through overlocking etc.

3. Minimal leverage
This is an exceptionally useful method. It uses the general principles of a combination of leverages and then a thrust, but whereas in the standard method the leverage is deliberately employed to supplement the thrust, in the minimal leverage method it is kept to an absolute minimum. It is used mainly as a means of placing a part in an available position and in an attitude of maximum relaxation. This places the contact point accessible for the thrust. The small amounts of leverage are arranged so that the joint is in as neutral a tension attitude as is possible; the accent is on the thrust, which has to be of a very high velocity if the forces are not merely to be dissipated in the tissues before the objective has been achieved. This is a particularly useful method where tension or torsion of the tissues is considered unwise, or in fact are impossible due to pain, contracture, apprehension, degeneration etc. This is the most delicate method of applying thrust techniques and is for some people almost impossible to master due to the accurate tension sense necessary. Unfortunately many manipulators never achieve adequate skill in this particular method mainly due to insufficient personal instruction. A great deal of meticulous practice is also necessary, but the effort is well worth while. The results which can be achieved are in excess of most other methods, and with far less trauma and after-treatment reaction. Separation of joint surfaces can be made to occur before surrounding tissues are put on full stretch and possible beneficial effects of joint cavitation with very small degrees of capsular stretch can be achieved. As an example, in a case of an acute disc prolapse it would not normally be possible to perform a normal type of full leverage technique. Any attempt to do so would be possibly traumatic as the torsion on the already damaged annulus might precipitate further prolapse. However using the minimal leverage technique it would be possible to achieve the separation of facets. Naturally in this instance the desirability of such a procedure would have to be carefully considered first as the pain response may not be invoked and one might be performing a technique which was contra-indicated for reasons other than pain.

4. Non leverage thrust
This is a type of thrust technique directed to a bony landmark such as a spinous process, without the use of leverage. This is more classically a chiropractic type of thrust technique, but in fact, most osteopaths also use some non-leverage methods in their approach to some conditions. Sometimes preliminary pressure in a particular direction substitutes for leverage and minimises the eventual amplitude of the thrust (see section on compression). This method requires either very high speed or very high force. Speed is preferable. Force often conceals weakness.

5. Non leverage thrust using momentum
The momentum effect in this technique is produced by applying and releasing the contact point pressure several times until a state of relaxation is sensed or until the momentum and oscillation of the tissues builds up adequate force at the contact point so that high application of force should not then be necessary.

Low Velocity Stress Techniques
These techniques use very low forces extremely slowly applied. They are often used with injunctions to relax and the operator is constantly taking notice of the patient's state of relaxation. They are often carried out with the use of respiration. They fall into four broad categories.

1. Low velocity stress using sustained leverage.

2. Low velocity stress using sustained traction.

3. Low velocity stress using sustained pressure.

4. Low velocity stress using articulation.

This terminology utilises our current trend to emphasise what is being applied but could cause confusion as these techniques are often given other names by other disciplines. Such terms as proprioceptive neuromuscular facilitation, neuro-muscular technique, functional technique, sustained release by positioning, counter strain, indirect release, muscle energy technique, disengagement techniques, ligamentous balance, fascial release and no doubt many others may come within this spectrum.

1. Low velocity stress using sustained leverage

In this method the operator holds the part in a so-called "corrective" position. An example of this would be a very lightly held combined leverage and thrust technique, but instead of a thrust, the position is maintained. The operator then slowly increases the position as the patient is encouraged to take deep breaths and is consciously asked to relax. The operator "listens" with his fingers and proprioceptive mechanism of his own joints and waits for the tissues to inform him that change has taken place. The other thing that may happen is that the operator may sense that a different pathway is necessary to achieve this feeling of relaxation and release of tissue tension.

Muscle Energy

Under this section we can also include isometric contraction techniques. These are called by a variety of names, including muscle energy technique, proprioceptive neuromuscular facilitation (P.N.F.), hold release, and no doubt other names. The guiding principle in these techniques is that the joint is taken up to a sense of barrier, usually in three separate planes. The patient is then instructed to attempt to push in the opposite direction away from the barrier. They therefore try to unwind themselves from the position. The operator resists the movement with an equal and opposite counter force and prevents any actual movement from taking place. This should not be allowed to develop into a wrestling match as the force necessary need never be very high.

The manoeuvre should not cause discomfort and it is important that the force is applied slowly and released slowly in conjunction with the patient's release. After a period of about three or four seconds of resisted contraction the patient is asked to relax slowly and the counter force is released at the same time. The joint is not forced against the barrier sense, merely held against it. A few seconds after relaxation has occurred the operator then slowly moves the joint further towards the barrier, which should have been found to have moved somewhat if the technique has worked. When this new barrier has been located the operator lightly pushes against it and then repeats the process. This is normally done three of four times. During all this the operator is sensing the existence of the barrier and being aware that it is a variable and looking for its progressive collapse.

What has been described is muscle energy technique using isometric contraction. There are two other varieties which are commonly used when this technique is considered. These are (a) isotonic contraction and (b) isolytic contraction. Isotonic contraction is used when the operator is attempting to increase tone in hypotonic muscles or muscles which have become inhibited for some reason. Naturally the effect which can be achieved where there is a neuropathy will be severely limited although there is sometimes more change than is expected. The same basic technique is used as in isometric contraction except that the muscle is allowed to contract in a controlled way and therefore the barrier is felt to move.

In isolytic contraction the aim is to break down severe adhesions and fibrosis in the muscle or muscles concerned. In this method the operator uses an amount of force just slightly greater than the patient's resistance to gently move towards the barrier. It should be noted that this last method can be very uncomfortable and should be used with care. In all these methods it is very important that the patient is informed what is expected of him and is asked to use only as much force against the operator as is comfortable. If this is not emphasised he sometimes tends to push too hard, produce pain and then is not keen to co-operate.

2. Low velocity stress using sustained traction

In this method traction, or sometimes a pressure so light as to be purely a disengagement, is applied very slowly and gently. This is done using the guide of the patient's respiration and by sensing the release of the tissues. This is often done with a little gentle, gradual movement into what is considered by the operator to be a more desirable position. Once again the operator tries not to impose his own impressions on the tissues but allows them to tell him what is their most comfortable direction of movement.

3. Low velocity stress using sustained pressure

This method uses the very slow application of pressure on a bony landmark, being applied very lightly at the outset, and slowly increased waiting for the relaxation of the tissues under the applicator, and may often be combined with some sustained positioning of the part in question. The velocity of application of force is of course very low and the force is increased slowly in time with respiration and the operator's perception of the tissues' relaxation. Naturally this method somewhat overlaps inhibition which was discussed in the section under rhythmic technique.

4. Low velocity stress using articulation

This type of approach can be divided into several different sub-headings: the first is really a fine sub-division of the previous categories utilising an extremely slow and gently applied oscillating movement at a rate which is never faster than about 14 cycles per minute and often slower according to the feed-back the operator is getting from the structures he is working on. So-called "functional technique" also comes under this head and cranial techniques could also be included here.

Functional Technique

This technique is a so-called "indirect technique" in that it does not utilise methods of finding a point of restriction or resistance to movement and forcing it into an opposite direction. In fact it uses exactly the opposite. Diagnosis of a textural abnormality in the tissues is made in the normal way with palpation. A gradient of abnormality can be felt in a particular area and the centre of this area is made a point of focus. The use of light tapping over the spinous process and para-vertebral tissues is brought into play also to emphasis areas which are particularly "different". This difference can best be summed up as the difference between tapping a hollow box and a solid piece of wood. The

hollow structure will have a resonance which is quite different from the solid one. The rate and depth of this type of tapping, which is performed with the fingertips, varies from operator to operator and patient to patient. With very little practice significant areas of difference can be identified. Subjectively, from the patient's point of view it is extremely easy to become aware of this "gradient" of difference.

Once the area of maximum difference has been identified one hand of the operator is used as a monitoring hand and keeps a constant palpatory awareness of tissue changes. The patient is asked to co-operate and allow himself to be gently moved whilst joining in this movement in a passive way. The part under the palpating hand will be felt to increase or decrease its sense of resistance as soon as any movement pathway is initiated. The important thing about this technical approach is that it is the initiation of movement which triggers off the response under the palpating hand. Each movement can be performed in a specific order and there will be an instant feed back of either "ease" or "bind". As this is an indirect technique the object is to find each direction of ease and add them together rather than using the principles of most direct technique, where in theory one is looking for directions of bind and forcing them to become free by the application of external force.

In functional technique all possible parameters of movement direction are utilised and the "ease" movements are summated, the idea being to produce an absolute situation of relaxation at the particular level concerned and therefore a reduction of tone and sensitivity at the part being palpated by the monitoring hand. As this is a somewhat subtle method, personal tuition is really essential as all parameters of movement have to be utilised and this is difficult to describe in writing. However, it is not difficult to understand the principles and it is included here for the sake of completeness. The common movements of flexion, extension, side bending to each side and rotation to each side are naturally used. Translatory movements of the body as a whole are also considered important in this method, the whole body being taken into an antero-posterior direction or a postero-anterior direction and a lateral direction to one side or the other, once again whichever is producing the maximum ease. The other aspect of this technique which makes it somewhat unique is the emphasis on the utilisation of response to respiration.

The patient is asked to start an inward breath and the palpating hand once again monitors if there is increasing or decreasing resistance. The same is done with expiration.

To summarise therefore, a functional technique applied to a particular vertebral segment will consist of (a) the operator finding the area of maximum tissues texture abnormality, (b) confirming this with gently tapping over the spine, (c) the patient will then be asked to co-operate in the movements which take place and the operator will use one hand to monitor and the other hand to move the patient in consecutive order into all the different directions of possible movement and include also response to respiration. The beauty of functional technique is that the part in question need never be taken to its full limit of movement in any one direction as the summation of these directions of ease are purely guided by the response to the initiation of movement and consequently the sense of relief which is achieved in the tissues is acquired in mid range. This is of course particularly useful in the hyper-acute case, the very nervous patient, or where it undesirable to use anything more than the gentlest possible techniques.

This method is rather difficult to grasp, particularly for experienced manipulators as it is somewhat different from methods that they may well be used to. However, its use should not be underestimated. The whole importance in the difference between these techniques and the other categories of rhythmic and thrust techniques is that the operator is constantly aware of subjugating his own ideas to a large extent and allowing the patient's structure to inform him as to what it needs by a feed-back mechanism. These are nearly all exceptionally gentle techniques. One is waiting for a response and answering that response with a minimum of imposition. A mastery of this type of technique introduces an extremely useful extra dimension to even conventional "hard" techniques because palpation is improved and tactile awareness is far more accurate and the rapidity in achieving the desired change in the structure is rewarded with better results.

One is therefore using gentler and gentler treatment which is not only less potentially traumatic, but is much less of a strain on the operator's own structure.

All these techniques are a form of inhibition, in that areas of irritability are quieted, the operator is constantly looking for the state of ease and release, rather than looking for the point of bind and barrier and attempting to fight through it.

Whilst it must be said that anybody can learn to manipulate, the fine details of these subtle types of techniques require constant assiduous practice to ensure their effectiveness. These methods sometimes produce a situation in which the patient considers that nothing is being done. This is particularly the case in patients who are experienced in being manipulated! The ensuing results will tend to nullify this but there is no doubt that some patients prefer "hard" methods. No one particular technical approach is the answer to all problems and the wider the spectrum of the operator's armament the more he is liable to be able to help a broader span of patients and a greater number of conditions with greater facility.

Cranial Techniques

Once again I feel that this subject needs the benefit of intense personal instruction to make a practitioner proficient. Nevertheless the principles can be stated simply and the reader is referred to specific texts elsewhere for the full background to this subject and further details.

The broad details of the guiding principles of cranial osteopathy can be listed under five headings.

1. The existence of an inherent motility of the central nervous system, i.e. the brain and spinal cord.

2. An inherent motility and pulsatile nature of the cerebro-spinal fluid.

3. The existence of reciprocal tension membranes, namely the meninges, particularly the falx cerebelli and the tentorium.

4. The mobility of the cranial bones around articular axes.

5. The mobility of the sacrum between the ilia.

To those not introduced to this concept these principles may seem rather unusual. However these are all palpable phenomena to the trained hand and have a certain amount of documented evidence of their existence.

The cranio-sacral rhythmic impulse can be felt throughout the body but is strongest when in contact with the cranial bones which are the vehicle through which these techniques are classically performed. A whole series of holds designed to influence different aspects of the above-named points have been worked out. These techniques utilise fine palpation and specific directions of forces. They can produce quite specific and sometimes spectacular results in a number of cases and they form a very useful addition to the categories of "reflex techniques". Some practitioners, when adept, can successfully treat many seemingly "orthopaedic" types of condition as well as purely local symptoms deemed to originate from cranial mechanism dysfunction.

MODIFYING FACTORS IN TECHNIQUE

All techniques are amenable to modifications and an attempt has been made to identify the most important modifying factors to enable the practitioner to choose as nearly as possible the type of technique for the individual case. Thus the morphology, age, sex, and general state of health of the patient can be taken into account. The modifications also make allowances for variations in size and skill of operator.

1. Force

This is probably the most important modifying factor when applying manual techniques as it relates the technique to the patient and his pathology. It can be sub-divided into light, medium, and heavy for recording purposes. The desirability of achieving the objective with the minimum of force has been emphasised already. Force stresses tissues. Stress can induce strain which can be defined as deformation within elastic limits. Deformation may lengthen, shorten, torsion, bend or compress tissues. Beyond the elastic limit there will be some form of damage.

To assess the breakdown of forces involved in a given technique, it is important to consider more than just pushing relatively gently or firmly on the contact point. There are many ways in which forces can be increased or decreased. Force in a thrust technique for example could be increased by one, several, or all of the following.

1. Increase of velocity, achieved by increase of speed of the operator's muscle contraction.
2. Increase of applicator weight. This is performed by the operator leaning more heavily on the contact point. This causes a preliminary deformation of the tissues.
3. Increase of leverage performed by altering the length or complexity of the leverage.
4. Increase of tension, this being a combination of all the varied factors which go to make up a particular technique.
5. Increased exaggeration of leverage which can be an alteration of its speed or its amplitude.
6. A late timing of thrust relative to the exaggeration of leverage.

7. An introduction of momentum into a thrust.

A careful consideration of all these factors will prove food for thought and several others to be varied should come to mind. Naturally a reduction of force could be achieved by a decrease of any of the above.

It can thus be seen that even an apparently simple matter such as force is made up of a whole mass of complexities. The actual application of force in pounds per square inch is limited by the weight of the operator whereas the variations governed by modifications allow small operators to increase force when necessary. A strong operator can manage most cases without having to introduce some of these factors; however, he may still meet his match in a very large or heavy patient and then strength is no substitute for skill.

The other modifying factors follow.

2. Amplitude

This refers to the distance traversed by the applicator when the leverage or thrust forces are applied. This is particularly important in thrust techniques, but many other procedures will also utilise variable amplitude to affect the depth of the treatment. An articulation technique could be performed at the limited range of flexibility of a particular joint to attempt to stretch intrinsic structures of the segment. Conversely it could be performed over a wide range to generally move all the tissues in a particular area. Amplitude could therefore be classified as short, medium or long. In a consideration of thrust techniques, the shortest possible amplitude is desirable to minimise excess stress on the tissues. Having said this at several points it should be noted that there are some occasions when a long amplitude thrust may be necessary to break through adhesions around a particularly chronic area of fibrosis.

3. Velocity

This refers to the speed of movement of the applicator, and once again is of particular relevance in thrust techniques. This is because the operator is relying on the build up of kinetic energy and the rate of movement will determine the amount of energy generated. Velocity helps to confine the force to a defined area or point. The high velocity, short amplitude thrust remains the classical osteopathic technique. Not all thrusts need be applied at ultra high velocity as the needs of the tissues vary. Some operators are unable to achieve very high velocity for various reasons. Providing they are aware of this they can modify their technique accordingly to achieve the desired result using alternative methods. Force in thrust techniques is built up by acceleration of the mass or weight of the applicator. The velocity and acceleration is the product of the operator's muscle contraction suddenly applied. The "knack" of this very rapid movement used in thrust techniques takes a variable time to learn. Some operators find no difficulty in acquiring it whilst others find it takes a considerable time. The key seems to be tied up in an ability to relax before the thrust. This comes from considerable practice and having confidence to carry through the manoeuvre without excessive hesitation. Hesitation before performing a particular technique leads to a tendency to fatigue in the operator's palpatory awareness and thus a loss of direction in the technique as well as the tendency to make the patient excessively uncomfortable. This does not mean that technique should be rushed but unnecessary delay in carrying out a procedure is to be avoided. When practising a given hold it is better to take up the position several times rather than holding the final position too long. This is not really a part of the actual velocity of the technique, but is nevertheless important to enable the operator to get to the actual effective part of the technique without wasting excessive effort. The part of the technique which does the work is not the taking up of the position, but is concerned with what is done when the position has been taken up.

4. Plane

This can be defined as the direction in which force is applied. Naturally this must relate to the anatomy of the part and also the objective of the technique. Force can be directed in a straight or a curving plane. It can be parallel or at a predetermined angle to the joint surface. This aims the force at a particular structure. When using thrust techniques it is particularly important to identify the direction of force accurately to minimise strain and increase the effectiveness of the procedure. The sense of "give" when the plane has been correctly located is quite a specific thing and even though two techniques may look the same, the one that is going to work best is the one in which the plane has been located most accurately.

5. Tension

This can be defined as the very subtle aspect of the application of leverage or stress and is made up of the combination of forces applied, and the creation of a situation in which the patient can relax. This must be combined with the placement of the part in an optimum position for the required technique.

Handling and positioning of the area are of particular relevance and sometimes several trial positions are required in order to reach the state of optimum tension. It should be noted that optimum tension is not necessarily maximal tension. All techniques can be carried out at high, medium or low tension. This is once again according to the needs of the structure, the state of the tissues and the desired effect. When the plane of a given joint is determined accurately, first by a knowledge of the anatomy and then by "playing" with the joint, the tension will not feel quite perfect until the joint is placed in the right position to achieve the cleaving or separating action. Variations in anatomy will be evidenced with the operator's fingers as leverage is applied if the tension sense is highly developed. The moment in the application of leverage or stress when a thrust or increase of leverage is applied determines the amount of tension in the tissues as well. This can be classified as synchronised, early, or late application.

Synchronised

This is the most usual method where a thrust or extra leverage is applied at the same time as the maximisation of the leverage or stress. By accident or design synchronised timing is not always achieved. Too early diminishes force, too late increases it.

Early

This is where the thrust or forces are applied slightly in advance of the maximisation of tension or leverage. This is a particularly useful method when the mobility of an area is very restricted due to spasm or degeneration. An excess of tension in such a case would cause premature locking or prevent relaxation through pain etc. As an example of this consider a typical cervical thrust technique performed on a pyknic morphology patient. Full locking and high tension would completely block the technique.

Using early tension takes more skill and practice, but an ability in this particular direction enables many cases to be treated which would otherwise be very difficult with "normal" synchronised tension. Using thrust techniques combined with minimal leverage, the joint never reaches its limit of travel in any direction. Those around it are not strained excessively and in the presence of osteophytes and other degenerative change, trauma is minimised.

Late

This is when the thrust or increase of force is applied slightly after maximisation of leverage. This will produce the maximum amount of stress, strain and mobilisation effect and is very powerful, particularly in thrust techniques. It does sometimes have a use in heavily built subjects providing adequate precautions are taken. Inadequacy of technical skill should not be compensated by excessive use of this modification.

6. Arrest

This is an aspect of a combination of amplitude and velocity, being the point at which the force is taken off. This is particularly important in thrust techniques, where the arrest is usually very abrupt for reasons already stated.

There are two main reasons for using an abrupt arrest. Firstly this helps to avoid stressing the tissues by going too far. Secondly, when using this method it is possible to send a "shock wave" through the tissues and produce a separational gapping of joint surfaces later than expected due to the deformation of tissues ahead of the thrust. This phenomena is highly developed in some of the chiropractic manipulative techniques. After the thrust the final position is held for a few seconds, partly to prevent reflex muscle spasm, and partly to utilise this shock wave effect at tissues remote from the actual thrust point. When using rhythmic techniques the arrest is likely to be of a much more graduated nature.

7. Onset

This term is used to describe the mode of application of force; it is usually graduated in rhythmic techniques or abrupt when using thrust techniques. The actual onset of application of force in a particular technique may of course be early or late in the application of leverage, so altering the level of comfort for the patient and this should constantly be considered to produce the maximum state of co-operation. A conscious attempt should be made to keep the tissues in a comfortable state until the last possible moment. The technique is then carried out and tension is let off thereby placing the part in as little tension, for as little time as possible.

8. Primary and Secondary Leverage

Where a leverage is built up by the use of two or possibly more positionings of a joint or area, there is always a primary or cardinal leverage which is the main direction in which the force is going to go. Secondary or further leverages generally serve to lock or stabilise the components of the technique and localise the force to a particular segment or segments. Success in manipulative technique is greatly enhanced by an accurate identification of all the component parts and an awareness of the direction of primary leverage to prevent application of the thrust to joints which are already locked by an over application of secondary leverages.

Not only will an excess of secondary leverage be uncomfortable for the patient but it will tend to reduce the effectiveness of the technique and thereby make the treatment less successful.

As a general rule the more parameters of leverage direction that are introduced into a given technique, the less the movement would be available in any one particular direction and sufficient "slack" must be left in the primary leverage direction to allow the tissues to absorb the force without producing jamming and overlocking and therefore unsuccessful technique.

Momentum techniques are sometimes discouraged because of the tendency to use excessive force or leverage. This need not apply providing an awareness of the difference between primary and secondary leverage is maintained. Holding the secondary leverage positions and only using the momentum in the primary direction is more liable to be successful and less liable to cause overlocking.

9. Contact Point Pressure

Where a thrust or force is to be applied to a small point or area, a certain degree of pressure of the applicator must be maintained on the contact point in order to secure a degree of accuracy and help limit amplitude. Because some of the "slack" of the tissues has been taken up by the contact point pressure the actual amplitude and force can be considerably less and also the correct plane of force can be more accurately determined.

There is a sense of "give" in the accurate direction for the thrust. When extreme pain or tenderness is encountered it may be impossible to employ firm enough contact point pressure and then it has to be increased only fractionally before the completion of the technique and removed immediately afterwards. This pressure should constantly slightly alter from one part of the applicator to another to maintain proprioceptive awareness and find exactly the correct force and plane.

10. Handling

This refers to the manner in which care is exercised in the placement of the hands on the patient having due regard for aesthetic considerations, avoidance of pain and discomfort, and an attempt to promote a state of maximal relaxation and confidence. This in turn will produce improvement in co-operation of the patient and therefore compliance of their tissues to help reduce the stress on them and the patient as a whole. A calm unhurried approach using warm hands and a sympathetic touch will go a long way to improving patient confidence. Another aspect of handling as distinct from actual avoidance of digging in nails, excessive grip and rough approach, is related to smoothness of delivery of technique. In general it should be possible to have some plan as to sequence of techniques in a particular treatment. This will only come with experience and practice but a little thought will save constantly turning the patient in acute pain, as one example. Blending one technique into another is an art which makes treatment much more comfortable and gives confidence to the patient. Rhythmic techniques lend themselves particularly well to this but the translation of a rhythmic technique into a thrust need not be any different. The term handling should also encompass the whole of patient to practitioner relationship and vice versa with regard to an awareness of pain perception and nervous reaction to the techniques being used. The sympathetic operator will keep his patient informed as to what to expect at any particular time during a treatment so as to avoid needless anxiety. This is particularly necessary when using thrust techniques for the first time on a patient who could understandably become alarmed if not suitably forewarned. Some operators seem to have a natural touch in this essential subject of handling whereas others need to be constantly on the alert for pulling of hair, digging in of fingers, pinching of skin and all the other common pitfalls.

The finest education in handling comes from being treated, worked on or practised on by one's colleagues. One knows immediately if the touch is able, or otherwise, and if one is able to relax or if undue tension is making the process more difficult for both parties. If a "fight" develops then there has to be a "winner" and therefore a "loser". Both parties working in the same direction is obviously preferable.

11. Positioning

Most techniques can be carried out in a variety of positions, e.g. sitting, sidelying, prone, supine etc. The thoughtful operator should try to find out the position in which the patient is most relaxed. The other chief consideration here is that the tissue or part to be worked on must be accessible so that the technique can be carried out in the most effective way.

This would depend on a number of factors such as the size and weight of the patient in relation to that of the operator as well as the acuteness or chronicity of the particular condition at that time. Techniques are available to deal with virtually all areas in nearly all positions. Some are more efficient than others and are to be preferred in most cases. Nevertheless a thorough knowledge of all possible positions for technique can be of great assistance in certain circumstances. For example a patient who was suffering from vertigo would far prefer to be treated in ths sitting position usually. In such a case, if the cervical region were to be worked upon, the supine position might produce an attack and therefore would be best avoided. The relative advantages of reduction of gravity promoting muscle relaxation would be outweighed by other considerations. If the operator is aware of tissue response he will on occasions have taken up a particular hold in a particular position and then have had to abandon the procedure and try another hold or position completely.

12. Use of Respiration and Injunctions to Relax

Many techniques are facilitated by the application of force at a given phase of respiration. This is most usually in exhalation. Patient relaxation will often be better if they are asked to inhale and exhale gently several times and the technique carried out towards the end of one of these exhalation phases. In general it is unwise to leave exhalation to its extreme as the patient is then just about to inhale and there will be very little recoil left in the tissues. If the technique were to be performed a little way before the end of respiration there would be a natural spring from the residual air. The relaxation achieved by exhalation serves the dual purpose of allowing the tissues to have some degree of spring, as well as distracting the patient.

Sometimes an injunction to relax at a particular point can be useful, and as previously stated, in some approaches, the active co-operation of the patient can be used to position the part in a particular way to assist the technique or take the patient's mind off what is being done. As an incidental point in some patients the word "relax" seems to cause problems and some alternative such as "let it go floppy" or "try and let me do the moving" or some similar request is often preferable. If the patient is being kept informed as to what is going on these injunctions are less often necessary.

13. Operator Stance

It is wise to make a constant study of one's own stance in order to minimise stress and strain on the operator's own structure. This will help to minimise fatigue and will improve the delivery of whatever technique is being performed. The improvement in proprioceptive awareness is considerable if the operator's own tissues are not on strain.

Analysing the way different techniques are performed can lead to some useful conclusions. As an example of this, in a thrust technique, the force is generated not purely from the hands, or even the hands and arms. In some techniques the hands and arms become relatively rigid, the whole pectoral girdle is seen to momentarily lock, and the operator's own spine is often placed in rotation usually with extension. This produces a rigid lever operating from the floor, through slightly flexed knees, a semi-rigid spine and a somewhat taughtened pectoral girdle. The longer the lever the less the force that needs to be applied to its end, and

therefore, if the operator's whole body becomes a long lever, the amplitude of force at the end need only be very small to produce the required result. As an example, consider a lumbar thrust technique sidelying, thrusting with the right hand on the patient's left gluteal region with the operator's left hand holding back on the patient's left shoulder. If the operator places his right leg behind his left and twists his own spine, in this case to the left, his own right shoulder, rotated spine and straight right leg will form a very rigid lever with which only a small downward force is necessary.

With only a slight flexing of the knees a high force can then be generated at the contact point. A common mistake when performing this type of technique is for the operator to drop his own spine into flexion which is potentially traumatic for him as well as being less effective in terms of the actual technique itself. The sharpness of arrest which was discussed earlier can be achieved much more easily with the operator's own spine being rigid for this short period of time. Conversely the smoothness and control necessary in articulatory techniques can better be achieved if the operator stands square to the patient and is then in a position to apply a more graduated arrest and onset of technique. Some techniques have to be carried out whilst standing on one leg and this is obviously less stable than whilst both feet are on the ground. Use of weight rather than muscular effort is always preferable and a careful study of operator position can help considerably to reduce strain. An adjustable table makes life much easier in this respect.

14. Operator Relaxation

There is an inherent tendency for the inexperienced operator to hold himself rigid. This mitigates against delicate work using accurate timing and tension sense. As stated in the last section, a rigid lever at the moment of thrust will assist the technique, but this rigidity must only be applied at the last possible moment. A conscious relaxation is often necessary to enable the operator's proprioceptive mechanism to accurately sense what is happening, and the tension can be accelerated at the last possible moment to produce the maximum effect. In patients who are exceptionally tense and will not allow the technique to take place without resistance, operator relaxation can be used as a specific part of the technique. If the operator consciously tenses into the technique and then relaxes, and then repeats this tensing and relaxing several times, the patient will soon join in with this rhythm. If the operator then rapidly reverses the direction in one of these phases when he appears to be relaxing and carries out the procedure it may catch the patient off guard and allow a successful technique to take place.

15. Compression

Using the principle of the lever, it is possible to apply a force through a long lever and the strength of the force is divided, and the distance travelled is multiplied by the ratio of the length of the long lever to that of the shorter one. This applies particularly in the use of compression, especially when performing thrust techniques. The compression acts as an extra locking mechanism to emphasise all existing leverages and thereby form the effect of longer levers as the joint in question is more firmly locked without the need for increased leverage. It is not just contact point pressure, nor is it just an exaggeration of leverages. It does not have to be compression of a disc, as it is just as effective in peripheral joints and those without a disc. In practice, if one applies a particular leverage in a chosen way up to a point of fairly full tension, and then, to increase patient comfort, lets off the tension until the joint is relaxed, any thrust at that point would have to be of a fairly long amplitude to reach that tension situation again. If, however, after letting off the leverage, one applies compression, the joint does not feel to the patient to be in such an extreme state of tension. The torsional strain will be less and they will be much more comfortable. If the thrust is then applied, the amplitude need only be very short as the "slack" has been taken up with the close packing of the tissues and not with uncomfortable torsion. When used on peripheral joints this is done with a squeezing action. This force of compression is applied by a combination of isometric contraction of the operator's own muscles and by the use of his weight through gravity. With advantage this method can be used as a momentum approach. The operator tenses and relaxes a few times before performing the thrust. To try and keep potentially dangerous aspects such as force and amplitude to a minimum this additional vector of compression is very useful.

To illustrate using a lumbar sidelying thrust again, with the patient lying on his right side in a position of contra-rotation, left shoulder pushed sightly back and pelvis rolled toward the operator, any thrust applied in this position will be ineffectual unless a long amplitude is used.

However, if the operator will apply a downward pressure to the patient's shoulder girdle and pelvis towards the table he will find that whilst this pressure is maintained, there will be very little if any further rotation possible and the joint will be placed on tension. The thrust can then be applied by the downward pressure rather than by increasing the rotation. To take this one step further, if the patient is placed in a position with even less rotation, but the compression force is increased, leverage amplification can be achieved with hardly any increase of actual leverage. This can be taken to the point where the leverage is almost nil and the effect of localisation is achieved with compression alone. This will inevitably produce some discomfort at the contact point in some cases due to heavy pressure. This can be minimised by using variable pressure and momentum. In fact the leverage is inversely proportional to the compression force.

This does not only apply in thrust techniques as articulatory techniques will be considerably more powerful and localised if this method of approach is used. Compression can be introduced also into soft tissue techniques. As an example with the patient prone, cross fibre kneading applied to the erector spinae muscles can be made much more effective using compression. If the operator will compress downward firstly and whilst maintaining this pressure, then apply the lateral pressure, it will be found that the effect is greatly amplified. The medial to lateral amplitude need then be very small and thus the distortion of tissues is also minimised. This incidentally does not need a great effort from the operator as his weight, not muscles, is doing the work. The full effect of using compression when performing thrust techniques seems to be threefold. The first effect is the one already mentioned of long and short lever amplification. The second is one of utilising a force which produces a state of greater relaxation in the muscles as one is "splinting" them and allowing them momentarily to relax. The third effect is related to certain types of indirect techniques. In some of these techniques such as cranial and functional technique, compression is sometimes used as a disengagement to allow tissues to have free play. This is sometimes in directions that they would not normally go without the releasing effect of the compression force. As an example, if a patient is placed in a sidelying position with the knees gently bent and one hand palpates the lumbar musculature whilst the other hand presses vertically downwards on the side of the pelvis, the lumbar muscles wll be felt to relax and tense in time with the increase and decrease of pressure respectively. By inducing small amounts of leverage and alterations in the direction of this pressure, the relaxation will be found to be greater or lesser and the optimum position can be found.

Most skilful manipulators utilise this approach to a greater or lesser extent, sometimes without necessarily identifying it as a particular parameter in their techniques. An attempt to utilise this and evaluate its usefulness can be a considerable help in improving technique efficiency. The use of traction is often advocated to reduce the chance of tissue damage, but this method of compression has been found to be much more effective in most cases.

16. Isometric Contraction

This forms another method of minimising force necessary, particularly in thrust techniques. Using this type of approach in combination with conventional thrust techniques, one can utilise the benefits of muscle energy technique in combination with more traditional methods. The operator can take up a given leverage in the usual way but then ask the patient to consciously fight back against that position and the operator then prevents the unwinding of the leverage firmly for some three seconds. He then asks the patient to relax simultaneously with the operator's relaxation. This can be repeated three or more times. If the patient is in the absolute optimum position for a particular thrust technique, during one of these repetitions, the joint in question will be felt to release. Even if this has not occurred, when retesting the movement range, there is often a considerable increase in range and quality of play. Even if there has not been any improvement in play, the operator can utilise the temporary rebound reflex relaxation in the muscles which will have occurred after the contraction to follow through the technique which was being performed in the first place. The thrust will then only need to be relatively gentle as the refractory period is active for a few seconds. This type of approach is particularly useful in the patient

who is prone to tense up anyway as one is using this tendency instead of it being a nuisance.

17. Resistance

When building up a leverage in some manipulative approaches, there is an insistence on engaging the barrier sense, and then applying an overpressure. Others will find the barrier and then move into the diametrically opposite direction such as in the usual approach to functional technique. In fact, in conventional direct techniques, the optimum position is a combination of both. The joint surface which one is hoping to move should be at the point of most tension to utilise the gapping effect. However the periarticular tissues, which in this case should usually not be tensioned excessively, are under as little tension as possible. This is assuming that the prime intention in the particular technique is to separate facets, rather than influence directly the surrounding tissues. If the intention is to produce maximum effect in the periarticular tissues then of course the opposite method will apply.

To achieve this balance between minimum and maximum resistance is often impossible, but on many occasions an active search for this delicate point of balanced resistance can be rewarding. Occasionally if an excessive leverage has been applied, the joint will be heard and felt to release as the patient is being unwound from the position. This will occur at a point of tension less than that at which the thrust was applied. If a conscious search for this point of minimum tension in surrounding tissues is made, this desirable situation can be achieved more often so that the joint in question can be coerced into a state of freedom rather than battered into submission. This requires very accurate tension sense, a constant awareness of tissue states and an alertness to the feedback mechanism to constantly slightly vary the pathway to the optimum. This is not possible if techniques are learnt as a series of procedures or movements. The plane of the direction of force will sometimes alter quite considerably during the execution of a technique. This is not really surprising since all joint surfaces are curved to a greater or lesser extent.

The current thinking on causation of joint fixation is coming down on the side of muscle action rather than any inherent bony fixation. If this is in fact the case then the function of joint manipulation is to affect the receptors in the joint mechanism rather than "unlocking" the joint. Certain situations of joint locking do undoubtedly occur, but in fairly rare cases as a sole entity. These situations seem far less important than the reflex pathways which surround most musculo-skeletal dysfunction. On this basis, the performance of thrust techniques should be primarily for the reduction of afferent input to the cord, and thereby reduce efferent outflow and so reduce embarrassment in the tissues caused by this state of hyperexcitability. Hence the current emphasis on minimal stress techniques rather than the more powerful long leverage forceful ones.

Experimental evidence of overaction of the gamma system with abnormal spindle function in the muscles affected, seems to be a reasonable basis of a working hypothesis at this time. If these theories are extrapolated, the type of manipulative procedure used is unimportant providing the result can be achieved as stated of joint release. Although on rare occasions specific directions of manipulation need to be considered, in general, positional factors are considered unimportant. This is at variance with the teaching of some authorities, as positional factors are considered paramount in various manipulative systems. If a great deal of time is spent in accurately analysing specific directions and positions of joints, the conclusion as to the direction that the particular technique needs will produce the same direction of least resistance in the periarticular structures, and maximal resistance in intraarticular structures that accurate palpation will deduce. It is postulated therefore that accurate palpatory assessment of joint function during technical procedures is as useful a guide to directions of force as is any preconceived notion about named lesion positions.

18. End Feel

If full use of minimal tissue tension, and delicate techniques is being utilised, there may well be occasions when despite evidence of joint separation, there is not the quality of "end feel" in joint range which is seen to be necessary. Movement quality may not be adequate and range less than expected. Another thrust may well be needed, possibly in a different plane, or with a slightly different amplitude or velocity etc. Any decision as to the need to reduplicate thrust techniques can only be made on the basis of experience but end feel awareness can be a useful guide. End feel of joint movement can be used as a premanipulation guide where the joint is placed in a "pre-thrust" position and tested for quality of end of range movement to give a clue to the type of procedure most likely to restore function. A "rubbery" resistive feel is generally a warning sign.

Synopsis of Approaches to Applying Osteopathic Techniques

1. Handling
The hands must always be placed gently and carefully on the patient. The patient must be encouraged to relax as much as possible by the demeanour of the operator. Unnecessary pain should be avoided and any procedure which is of an unaesthetic or embarrassing nature should be avoided if possible. Good handling consists of smooth transition from one technique to another without jerky movement and in a planned approach.

2. Positioning of patient
This should generally be performed slowly and purposefully. If necessary one can try several different positions for a given treatment until the patient and operator feel as relaxed as possible. For every technique there are several alternative positionings which make the procedure more or less effective. It makes sense to find the best one.

3. Posture of operator
The operator should consider at all times their own posture from the point of view of reducing fatigue and possible injury to their own structure as well as maintaining a good balance to prevent excessive force being applied to the patient. This will improve efficiency, lessen fatigue, and is of particular importance in any technique where the operator is taking some of the weight of the patient.

Small, light operators of both sexes become extremely proficient at utilising leverage as distinct from weight when performing technique. In learning technique it is a good idea to have some instruction from small operators to help acquire skill in this facet of manipulative methods. Large operators can often get away with using their size and weight, but when they meet a larger than average patient, they may find that strength is no substitute for skill.

4. Weight taking

It is wise to reduce to an absolute minimum any techniques which involve taking the patient's weight. On occasions there is no other way, but if the table can be made to do most of the work physical stress can be minimised. Mechanical assistance in the way of hydraulically adjustable tables, pillows, straps etc. can often be used. Whenever the patient is capable they should be encouraged to turn themselves on the table, and a surprisingly little assistance from the operator can facilitate this.

5. Operator relaxation

It is advisable to be constantly aware of the necessity to relax when performing osteopathic treatment. A state of tension not only transmits itself to the patient and their tissues, but reduces the appreciation of palpation, leverage, pressure, stretch and other sensory perceptual factors. Fatigue is also increased if the operator is tense during treatment. This does not mean that techniques can be performed in a sloppy fashion, but a conscious attempt to promote an air of relaxed confidence will promote far greater co-operation from the patient.

6. Holds

The hand placement for a given technique can be varied in several different directions. The thoughtful operator should attempt not to grip excessively with the fingertips and this should be instilled very early in the training, although it is difficult when performing unfamiliar techniques to concentrate on all aspects of handling. It is a good idea to constantly re-evaluate the approach to any particular technique as the method which has become most comfortable by frequent usage may not be the most effective. Most operators restrict themselves to a relatively limited range of techniques, and can have great difficulty when called upon to perform in a different way.

7. Apparatus

It is often useful to experiment with different types of apparatus such as pillow, stool and plinth height etc. As already mentioned an adjustable plinth is extremely useful to achieve perfect balance with the variety of areas to be worked on. A rising head-piece is of some help in some cases, but suitable size pillows can be substituted. There are advantages and disadvantages in different widths of plinths. Patients feel more comfortable on a plinth of approximately 28 inches width. Unfortunately this width is not very practical for sitting astride techniques. It is also not very practical for techniques where the patient is sitting across the table as they will still be some distance from the operator even with their knees against the edge. This will mean that the operator will have to perform such techniques in a bent position which is obviously not a good idea. A compromise can be achieved by having a table which is fairly wide for half of its length, and then a taper toward the foot end for these astride techniques. The padding should be of sufficient density that it is not possible to "bottom out" and yet be soft enough to be comfortable and absorb some impact to help prevent injury. This is particularly necessary in prone techniques where the costochondral junctions are at risk. A table which is too firm can be counteracted by placing a pillow under the patient's abdomen in such a case. Ideally the plinth should be padded right over the edges so that the operator's thighs can rest against the edge to increase leverage when necessary. This also reduces discomfort for the operator if they are leaning on the edge to get close in for a particular technique. If the patient's leg or arm is placed over the side they will also prefer this to be padded.

8. Approach

The operator should cultivate an unhurried, calm, reassuring approach to the patient, particularly the very nervous, the aged and children.

9. Planning

It is not a good idea to give casual, off the cuff, unplanned treatment.

Empirical treatment will tend to have very mixed results. It is better to have an objective in mind based on a diagnosis, with some idea of a prognosis.

The thoughtful operator should be considering the immediate and long term objectives of the techniques which are being performed. A planned treatment avoids unnecessary turning over and over for the patient who may be in great distress when performing rotational movements. Unless there are specific reasons for a particular approach it is generally better to work towards a part in pain or discomfort rather than attacking it directly. Notwithstanding this a thorough palpatory investigation of the site of discomfort is reassuring for the patient and can give useful clues as to the types of techniques most likely to be effective to influence the affected tissues. Insufficient force to achieve the required result can be remedied by a reduplication of the technique using a graduated approach until the result desired is gained. Much experience is required to judge just the right degree of force in a given patient and it is always better to be ineffectual than dangerous. An ineffective technique can be repeated whereas one that causes damage may be disastrous. It is unwise to persevere with any technique, particularly a thrust technique, in the presence of extreme pain or resistance. Similarly if the patient is unable to relax there may be concealed pathology or anomaly and it is preferable to defer treatment or try some other approach. Specific contra-indications to manipulative technique are discussed in the next chapter.

10. Reactions to previous treatments
A feedback from the patient as to reactions will give considerable guidance to the advisability of continuing treatment or making a reassessment. Reactions out of proportion to those expected should always give cause for a re-evaluation. Like any other medicine, manipulative treatment has to be given in correct dosage. An overdose will cause adverse reactions whereas undertreatment may well be unable to produce the desired symptomatic and objective changes. It is nevertheless a far more common mistake to overtreat than to undertreat. If in doubt hold back.

Due to muscle "memory" it is often necessary to repeat a given procedure on subsequent occasions.

It is therefore unwise to attempt "miracle" treatments in one go. Making allowances for variations in fitness, resilience, sensitivity, and state of general health, different patients will react differently on various occasions. An accurate record of techniques carried out will give a useful reference on a subsequent occasion if there has been a severe reaction to treatment.

The interval between treatments is often of critical significance. The decision as to the spacing of treatments is only arrived at by a consideration of all the relevant factors relating to the chronicity, acuteness, urgency and of course practical factors of distance and advisability of travel etc. If a patient reports benefit out of all proportion to the techniques applied and therefore the expectation of result, it is generally wise to suspend any further treatment for a while as it is often possible to reverse the situation and regret not having paid heed to this simple instruction.

11. Types of thrust technique
On the basis of diagnostic data and pre-thrust trials, a pre-selection of technique will choose the approach most likely to succeed in a particular case. Osteopathic technique employs no follow through when using thrust technique and the short amplitude high velocity thrust remains the classical method of approach in suitable cases. Low force, accurate direction and a sympathetic feel for the tissues distinguish the efficient technician.

CONTRA-INDICATIONS

There is almost no treatment that is without some possibility of producing harm. The likelihood of causing damage with osteopathic techniques is small and with sufficient care can be reduced to the absolute minimum.

Contra-indications fall into several categories.

One useful way of looking at these is to consider them as (a) absolute and (b) relative. Absolute contra-indications will be considered under five separate headings.

1. Where manipulation could damage a bone already weakened by some pathological process.

2. Where there is evidence of severe nerve pressure such as cord or cauda equina signs.

3. Where there is evidence of circulatory disturbance from reflex arterial spasm or direct pressure.

4. Where the diagnosis is unsure.

5. Where pain or resistance prevents accurate positioning for the technique for any reason.

1. Bony Structure

Weak bony tissue
Bone can be weakened by a number of different pathological entities. Most of these can be seen on X-ray, but unfortunately symptoms may well be produced before the condition becomes evident radiologically.

Precise history taking and examination should help in the clinical judgement and assessment in all cases to illuminate as far as is possible the correct type of approach to each individual. Osteopaths have been justifiably criticised in the past for not making enough use of X-rays, although it has to be admitted that some of this reluctance has been based on a desire to save the patient unnecessary extra expense and radiation if they have already had hospital films done. It is hoped that with increasing co-operation between the professions, sharing of results of X-rays etc. can become more common. Infectious conditions of bone and neoplasms of a primary or secondary type will usually produce a symptom picture which is out of proportion to the signs.

This unexpected finding should always be a sign which puts the thoughtful operator on his guard and shows the need for further investigation. If the patient is obviously ill as well as in great pain, or if the muscle spasm is greater than that which one usually finds with normal musculo-skeletal conditions, the diagnosis should be thoroughly re-evaluated before any attempt at treatment is attempted. Advanced osteoporosis shows typical clinical signs but even in the absence of these no great attempts to "correct" areas of obvious deformity are ever wise. Absence of local signs of dysfunction, despite acute pain, warrants great caution.

2. Neurological

Spinal cord or nerve pressure syndromes
Where there is any evidence of cord pressure, particularly in the cervical column, where the room for the cord within the spinal canal is least, then thrust work is absolutely contra-indicated. This does not mean that in the same patient, some other part of their structure could not be successfully treated without damage. Where there are cauda equina signs or evidence of neuropraxia, it is generally wiser not to treat the patient anyway as these syndromes sometimes get worse regardless of what is done, and no charge of wrongful treatment could then be levelled. The case history, followed by even a cursory examination, should make this sort of condition very evident.

3. Vascular

Danger of circulatory damage
Osteopaths have an enviable safety record considering the possibility of damage when applying forceful manipulative techniques, particularly in the neck. The reason for their good record is most probably because the techniques they employ are generally considerably gentler than those of other disciplines. Nevertheless cases of severe arteriosclerosis are particularly susceptible to possible damage from over-vigorous manipulative methods. This is also true where there are certain anatomical abnormalities, once again particularly in the upper cervical area. There are various tests which have been devised to assure the least possible chance of damage when manipulating the cervical column. They are all methods of verifying the integrity of the vertebro-basilar system. No

series of tests can serve as a universal guide, but they do help act as a reasonable, reproducible system.

Extension test
With the patient seated, the examiner stands behind and slowly brings the patient's head into extension and then side-bends and rotates it, first to one side and then to the other. Any evidence of dizziness, nystagmus or dysarthria should cause the operator to abandon all attempts at thrust techniques and lead to an investigation of the reason for this postural hypotension type of symptom.

Hautant's test
With the patient seated and both arms stretched out in front of them at the same height, they are asked to close their eyes, and the head is moved into extension, side-bending and rotation as in the previous test. If one arm sinks and pronates this denotes evidence of impaired circulation.

De Klejn's test
In this test the patient lies supine with maximum extension of the head and the examiner is able to passively increase the extension, sidebending and rotation range and text for production of symptoms.

Flexion test
If extreme cervical flexion produces symptoms of paraesthesia, particularly in the lower limbs, then the possibility of a cervical bar should always be considered. A spondylotic bar can occur in patients of a generally younger age group than normal generalised spondylosis and this simple test should always be performed before cervical techniques are carried out.

4. Diagnostic

Lack of diagnosis
Manipulation of even the gentlest variety is best avoided until at least some sort of diagnosis or assessment has been arrived at. The possibility of hidden anomaly or pathology should always be considered. Empirical approaches will at best give inconsistent results, and at worst could be disastrous. Because it is possible to get a measure of success with empirical treatment, there is a tendency in certain quarters to learn "recipes" for techniques based on a list of findings. Although the experienced practitioner can often "get away" with this it is not to be encouraged as it leads to overconfidence and a tendency to disregard warning signs. Unfortunately the body is so ready to respond to manual therapy, often with surprising results, that a degree of pure empiricism, or working by rote tends to creep in.

5. Symptomatic

Pain and resistance
In the presence of pain and resistance in excess of that expected for that type of technique being utilised, a re-evaluation of the signs and symptoms should be considered. The less the experience of the operator, the greater the need to consider the absolute contra-indications to particular techniques. With increasing experience it is possible to be able to make some of these absolute contra-indications fit into the next category of relative contra-indications.

Before considering these it is evident from a perusal of the tests in this section that most of the classical tests designed for the protection of the vertebral arteries involve extremes of the combined movements of extension, side-bending and rotation. If these movements are capable of provoking arterial embarrassment, then it makes sense to avoid them when performing therapeutic techniques. The few tragedies which have occurred with cervical manipulation, not I hasten to add by osteopaths, have all been with excess use of extension, side-bending and rotation and then the superimposition of excess force. Because of this the current emphasis at the B.S.O. is on techniques with minimums of these potentially traumatic leverages.

6. Relative Contra-indications
Under this heading could be included a complete list of pathologies that may affect bone, disc, ligament etc. Any patient who has a particular pathology may also as an incidental matter have mechanical dysfunction with spinal segments. As long as the objective of the technique is to deal with the mechanical disorder, and suitable caution is taken, then any contra-indications in that case may be considered only relative. The reason for grading osteopathic techniques into their different varieties and different modifications, is that it should be possible to make a prescription of a particular approach to technique which would suit a given patient. Although a full combined leverage and thrust technique using high force, high leverage and long amplitude would be contra-indicated in an 80 year old with a stiff neck, that does not mean that very light,

delicate minimal leverage thrust techniques or muscle energy techniques could not be carried out in such a case.

Relating the technique to the physique, age, general health, and particular state of the tissues at the time is part of the diagnostic process and forms part of every pre-technique assessment.

Adverse reactions to previously carried out treatment of other types, or previous osteopathic treatment should put the practitioner on his guard as to either excessive sensitivity of the patient or their tissues. This may be due to some unforeseen reason or purely a patient with a low pain threshold. The latter is a very real entity and the warning signs of an excessively emphasised history and reaction to apparently minor symptoms, should lead to extreme caution. This tendency can be due purely to fear and distress, or in some cases, a tolerance to pain which is less than average.

If suitable care is taken to grade the treatment from the lightest possible forces, and only increasing the force according to the needs of the case, then the chance of adverse reaction and over treatment and damage is minimal. If however, despite these precautions, extreme reactions are encountered, a really thorough re-examination must be carried out to try and ascertain the reason if possible to prevent a recurrence. In many cases a severe reaction can be settled down by a confident statement that no damage has occurred based on a thorough examination. Despite the most meticulous care, the odd severe reaction to treatment in general, or particular techniques can occasionally occur. There are many methods of reducing the effects of adverse reactions. Some practitioners advise rest and heat, others advise analgesics or anti-inflammatories. Some osteopaths will apply simple massage techniques and yet others will carefully repeat the treatment plan previously applied. This latter on the basis that the tissues are just showing evidence of change and that they may as well get the full advantage by producing a major change anyway. My own approach is to examine the patient thoroughly using examination procedures which are basically treatment manoeuvres and try to find the reason for the reaction. If there is an area of inflammation or congestion, then apply gentle techniques, particularly of the "reflex" type to attempt to settle this, and then ask the patient to report in a couple of days either by telephone or in person. The mere fact of making contact seems to defuse the situation and restore the patient's confidence.

As was stated under the section dealing with dosage, the interval between treatments can be critical. A severe reaction may well settle in a day or two to a considerable improvement in signs and symptoms. If that same patient was seen during that phase of soreness from treatment, the practitioner might have wrongfully assumed that he had done the wrong thing, or had overdone what was done. For this reason, daily treatment is generally to be discouraged unless the operator is prepared to perform only minimal treatment on each occasion and is ready to accept the possibility of severe reactions by working on tissues which have not settled down from previous attention. Having said this, there are cases when for reasons of urgency, more frequent treatment may be essential. From experience I would say that in these cases absolute specificity is important. Short, purposeful treatment, aimed at doing only one thing on each occasion, is generally best.

The vexed question as to whether manipulative techniques should be used in the presence of evidence of disc prolapse will probably be the subject of discussion and argument for some time. In the author's experience, providing there are no signs of extreme nerve pressure, either before treatment, or whilst applying the technique positions slowly, then disc prolapse is a sign for caution not for abandonment of technical procedures. Powerful rotary techniques in the presence of X-ray evidence of large osteophytes are best avoided for fear of nerve impingement. Forced flexion techniques are unwise where there is evidence of disc prolapse in the lumbar spine as increase of prolapse can occur.

A joint which is obviously acutely inflamed is best left to rest for some time before treatment commences. Over zealous attempts to force a joint to free in this situation will lead to extreme reactions. The timing and selection of when to treat can only be gained by experience. Any patient who is obviously ill in a general sense needs either the lightest of approaches or leaving alone until they are better in themselves for their tissues to accept benefit.

Further relative contra-indications
During pregnancy, any technique which might jeopardise the health of the mother or developing infant should obviously be avoided. The chief danger of producing a spontaneous abortion occurs in the first trimester. In a patient with a history of

repeated abortion, any treatment should be withheld until after the three-month barrier. Treatment during the later stages of pregnancy will necessitate techniques modified from normal methods. The presence of hormonal relaxation of tissues makes most osteopathic procedures much easier and in fact light techniques can be very effective, and of considerable benefit. With sufficient care a pregnant patient can be treated right through her pregnancy, and in certain circumstances gentle osteopathic treatment during parturition itself can be of assistance.

X-ray evidence of calcification of the aorta is not in itself a total contra-indication to treatment, although it would of necessity mean that caution is essential. The possibility of damage to the structure is minimised if techniques using extremes of movement in any direction are avoided. In general, patients with this type of pathology would be of an age group where extreme rotation is best avoided anyway.

The existence of spondylolysis and spondylolisthesis is not necessarily a reason for witholding treatment. If the patient's symptoms are referable directly to the spondylolisthesis and there are cord signs, then osteopathic techniques of any degree of force are best avoided as there is a chance of causing further damage. However, many cases have a spondylolisthesis as an artefact, and its existence does not preclude the use of osteopathic technique. Techniques which are specific and are applied to the adjacent joints which may be a source of symptoms can be used providing enough skill has been acquired. Recent work has shown that traumatic onset spondylolisthesis can in many cases be a stress fracture of the pars interarticulares and therefore the treatment for this is immobilisation as in any other stress fracture. This has been shown to produce healing of the fracture site, therefore techniques of mobilisation in these cases are contra-indicated.

Conditions such as ankylosing spondylitis and Reiter's syndrome etc. are best not treated by manual methods in the active inflammatory state as it is possible to aggravate the situation. There is also a chance of rupturing the already disrupted ligamentous structures. This does not mean that the lower force techniques are contra-indicated necessarily.

There are several conditions which can weaken ligamentous structures, the most notable of these being rheumatoid arthritis. The gross destruction of peripheral joint capsules and ligaments is well known, but rheumatoid arthritis has also been shown to weaken the transverse alar ligaments. If thrust techniques are performed in the neck, particularly the upper cervical spine, in such cases a tragedy could occur and these techniques should be completely avoided.

Long-term use of steroids, particularly in high doses, can have the effect of producing osteoporosis, but can once again weaken ligaments and the transverse ligament retaining the dens is vulnerable. Long-term use of anticoagulant therapy sometimes leads to a similar situation. A patient who is taking these drugs will by the sheer nature of their condition also have atheromatous plaques. Any techniques which could disturb these, such as very vigorous mobilising by articulation technique or the use of powerful thrust techniques, particularly in the neck, are therefore best avoided in such a case.

Extreme scoliosis, particularly where there are organic changes evident with the consequent alteration in the shape of the vertebra and fibrosis of ligamentous tissues, would make accurate examination and assessment even more important than usual. The possibility of the presence of large osteophytes in such a case should be considered and X-ray is advisable before anything other than the gentlest of techniques is performed.

The other major consideration in such a case would be the advisability of disturbing the patient's adaptation to their shape and a careful assessment should be made bearing this in mind.

In a similar vein, very advanced spondylosis or other degenerative changes should direct the thoughtful operator towards certain categories of technique and away from others. Only experience can guide the operator in the prescription of dosage in any given case but it is always better to err on the side of safety. It is better to expect the worst possible condition and be wrong than to expect everything is all right, and be wrong!

Patients who have very severe diabetes are liable to have extreme reactions to osteopathic treatment and possibly incur disturbance of their insulin balance. Providing one is aware of this possibility and has warned the patient then normal treatment can be carried out.

In any patient where there has been a previous history of malignancy, the most thorough and searching examination should be carried out to be able to come to an accurate diagnosis as to whether the patient's symptoms are of a mechanical or pathological nature.

A sense of lack of "give" in the area when performing a particular technique should always be a warning to the operator that perhaps either the wrong technique has been selected, or that there is some hidden pathology or anomaly. Pressing on regardless in the hope that it will come right is not to be advised. Experienced operators can become very adept at diagnosing anomalous structures, and describing their shape and configuration without the use of X-rays. This may surprise many practitioners from other fields, but an accurate developed palpation sense makes this possible.

Any patient complaining of vertigo is liable to have the condition made worse by over vigorous treatment, particularly when applied to the cervical region. Some types of vertigo are amenable to osteopathic treatment but large amounts of rotation to the upper cervical spine can provoke an attack. This does not preclude the use of gentle techniques, avoiding the use of rapid head movements and avoiding having the patient lying too flat.

Psychological dependence on manual therapy is not uncommon and providing the operator has assured himself that the patient does have a true physical cause for his symptoms, then treatment can be valid. It must be said nevertheless, that patients of this type can become very good at emphasising their minor physical disturbances, and the inexperienced practitioner can become very involved with them, and find that it is very difficult to extract themselves from the dependency which develops. The problem hinges on deciding the importance of the inevitable physical signs which any spine manifests, particularly in a tense individual. It is a natural desire of any practitioner to help their patient, but allowing the patient to orientate their neurosis around their spine means that any physical therapy is doomed to failure.

Another category of patients in whom manipulative technique is relatively contra-indicated are those who have been treated very recently by another practitioner. The decision as to the choice of interval between treatments should be part of the pre-technique assessment. Tissue reactivity varies enormously from one patient to another, and it is a bigger mistake to over-treat than to undertreat. Excessive frequency of treatment can lead to a vicious circle. It is a mistake to treat the patient just because they are there. If their tissues are not ready for it, they are best left alone. A patient who has seen another practitioner recently may be unsatisfied, for various reasons, with the result. A reasonable period must be allowed for any reaction to settle down, and any benefit to accrue. If the practitioner is persuaded against their better judgement to treat the patient, a severe adverse reaction can be elicited due to a poor appreciation of the true tissue state which may be different due to the previous practitioner's treatment. The patient may be genuinely dissatisfied with the treatment they have received elsewhere, they may be playing one off against the other, or there may be some very good reason for their lack of response. All these factors need to be taken into consideration before starting on any treatment plan.

There is a widely held belief in some quarters that the use of high levels of traction will render all manipulative procedures "safe" as joint surfaces are separated, foraminae are opened and the chance of nerve or blood vessel impingement is reduced. It is dangerous to place absolute reliance on this although it is certain that in some cases, particularly when using violent techniques, it may be true. Traction, in its many guises, is a valid and useful method of treatment, but to use it to render safe an otherwise unsafe procedure seems an inadvisable approach. Excessive reliance on any absolute rule such as this is responsible for a rigid approach, with no possibility of variation in varying circumstances. The osteopathic approach is to make constant subtle changes according to the needs of the tissues at the time they are being worked.

An important relative contra-indication is in a case where the signs and symptoms do not seem to match. All experienced practitioners develop a "sixth sense" for situations they should not be dealing with. This a combination of experience, hunch, assessment and various other imponderables. If in doubt it is best to wait until further investigations have been performed. It is better to suspect the worst, and be wrong, than not to suspect anything, and be wrong.

PRINCIPLES OF LOCKING

Methods of producing locking to localise a force to a particular point or area have been arbitrarily taught in the past using the terms "ligamentous" and "physiological" locking. These terms are little used now as the method of producing locking or stabilising is seen to be less important than the result. The term "ligamentous" referred to the use of tension in tissues to produce the effect of localisation. Conversely the term physiological locking referred to the fact that when any spinal segment was placed in a position of rotation in one direction and side-bending to the other side, any force applied would tend to maximise at the apex of one of these levers.

In actual practice both of these methods are used at the same time. A thoughtful operator will use the combination of several complex leverages to position a part in an optimum placing so that only a slight emphasis of leverage will achieve a focus at the desired point. Locking need not consist of a steady "wind up" to a point and then the application of overpressure. This is of necessity very uncomfortable for the patient. An absolute point in which the forces come together needs to be found, but if this can be done without actually applying the necessary leverage until the last possible moment, the patient will feel more relaxed and therefore better able to co-operate with the procedure. This can only be done by the operator being aware of the feel of tissues which are just "off tension" so that he can tease the tension point by repeatedly approaching it from several slightly different positions until the absolute optimum can be sensed. The technique can then be carried out with great rapidity, and although the patient has been held at say 80% tension for some time, the last 20% is only applied for a split second. This needs the ability to palpate a pathway of resistance rather than an absolute position. To try to put into words the difference between locking "up to" a particular part of the spine as against "down to" that part is almost impossible. The intersegmental changes taking place when for example flexion is applied to an area as distinct from extension will govern which part of a given joint will be stressed by a particular technique. The influence of pathological or distorted physiological processes of degeneration and anomaly have to be considered at all times. These will produce distorted patterns and altered quality of movements, particularly at the extremes of range.

The physiological movements of the spine are such that most manipulative technique requires the utilisation of composite levers to achieve the stabilisation necessary to localise force. Almost all techniques can be performed with a variety of leverages. Let us assume a particular technique needs 30 degrees of flexion, 60 degrees of rotation and 20 degrees of side-bending.

If the flexion is applied first, there will be a tendency to put in greater than 30 degrees. The technique will still work but it will be found that the other levers have been decreased by the same amount as the flexion has been increased. Conversely if the rotation is put in first, it will tend to become the executive part of the technique. This interesting phenomena can be utilised consciously by constantly playing with all parameters of the combination of levers until the absolute optimum is found. Experienced operators usually apply any given leverage as a composite movement and are constantly varying the quantity of all the directions as the tissues yield or otherwise in each direction. In this way locking does not become full leverage and overpressue but achieves the desirable situation of being in as near a neutral position as possible until the critical time when the technique is finalised as an arc of movement rather than as an absolute position.

The principles of using a variety of different levers to produce a situation of localisation of force is referred to as locking. In the true sense, nothing is in fact locked, but the forces are concentrated more at one point than any other if this procedure is performed correctly. Extreme movement in any direction followed by an overpressure will stretch and deform tissues and could lead to damage if applied over vigorously. Utilising the locking process allows the force to be localised without any lever reaching its maximum range although the primary lever is usually taken further than all others.

The most common method uses a process of rotation to one side in the spine and a side-bending direction to the other side. The addition of small degrees of flexion, extension, compression, traction etc. will further aid the localisation. The way any particular operator builds up the levers to a given technique will of course vary from patient to patient and from one operator to another. Nevertheless the guiding principles obey certain ground rules. As a general rule any particular area of the spine can be manipulated using thrust techniques in a whole variety of positions and ways, although there are certain directions which will be the most effective, least traumatic and most comfortable for the patient. One useful guide is that locking can be produced quickest when using the movement least available in that particular area. The greater the range of possible movement, the more variety of locking procedures can be employed with relatively similar efficiency. To try and clarify this, consider the mid cervical spine. This area has a wide range of flexibility in most directions in the normal subject and so will be possible to position in most combinations of position for techniques to be performed although local morphological variations will sometimes vary this. However the lower cervical spine, due to the variation in the facet angles has less range of movement, particularly into extension, and therefore locking using flexion as a part of the leverage build-up would require much more range or movement than the use of extension.

Similarly in the upper cervical spine the movement least available, and therefore the one which will produce the most efficient and quickest locking without using large ranges of movement, is side-bending.

Having identified this principle it is not difficult to evaluate the particular directions that this theory will support for each area. Having said that, they all need a combination of side-bending and rotation to the other side, so-called "reverse rotation"; the other directions most efficient are as follows.

Upper Cervical—emphasise side-bending, although neck as a whole can be either in flexion or extension.

Mid Cervical—all positions possible therefore balance between directions emphasising rotation as it produces least discomfort.

Lower Cervical—emphasis on extension in addition to main leverages needs least range although extreme flexion is also effective.

Upper Thoracic—emphasis on extension and the rotation elements of movement locks quickest.

Mid Thoracic—depending on the degree of kyphosis, usually extension with side-bending.

Thoraco-Lumbar—extension produces quickest locking although extreme flexion is just as effective if more uncomfortable.

Mid Lumbar—neutral as this is a free moving area, emphasis on rotation produces best effect.

Lower Lumbar—due to the variation in facet angles this area is fraught with difficulties in trying to make general rules. However side-bending applied first, followed by the rotation element using flexion in the lordotic spine and extension in the flat spine will usually be effective.

Any general principles such as these are of course open to criticism, but the analysis of the idea behind this way of looking at locking can be used as a guide and starting point in the development of personal approaches to individual methods.

It must be pointed out that rotation to the right from above is the same movement as rotation to the left from below. This may seem self-evident but if this fact is considered carefully, it can alter the approach to a particular technique, and possibly make it effective where it would not be otherwise. The focussing of forces to a specific point, in a comfortable way for the patient and operator, is the essence of skill in manipulative technique. If a particular combination of leverages is applied in a progressive way to a point of full tension, not only will the patient be uncomfortable, but also the operator will probably be in a less than optimum position for efficient completion of the technique. However, if the build-up of tension is sensed, and the absolute point of tension is "teased" and approached from several different angles, and allowed to decrease, there will be a better appreciation of the optimum point at which the final force needs be applied. This "playing" with the joint is not a vague movement but needs to be a considered variation of all the components of directions of movement possible in a constant attempt to achieve the desired sense of release using the position which stresses the structure as little as possible. It does take time and practice to be able to identify the optimum directions of force without the guidance of full tension. The time taken to acquire this skill is well worthwhile in production of quicker results, and less adverse reactions to treatment. If this method of approach seems completely intangible at first, it is better to carry out technique using full leverages and gradually refine the method, introducing these principles as experience, and appreciation of the principles accumulates. It is all to easy for experienced practitioners to fall back on methods which although effective, are procedural and of necessity limited in the benefit they can produce. The beauty of the osteopathic approach using the infinite variety of possible composite levers and directions is that there are no absolutes and therefore nearly all situations can be catered for.

APPLIED TECHNIQUE

Pure technique is an interesting academic exercise but has little use in application to real patient situations. The adaptation of basic techniques to create a particular influence on a named tissue or tissues is the basis of applied technique. If the concept of creating change in a particular tissue, rather than executing a sequence of movements is considered, then real life situations can be dealt with. For this a full understanding of the purpose of particular movements needs to be grasped. Using the principles of physiological movement possibility in a given part it should be possible to devise techniques within certain limits which differ from the classical ones but are none the less effective.

Consideration must be given to selection of techniques to modify particular physiological processes, influence pathological states and modify body mechanical functions. Techniques chosen should be suited not only to the local tissue to be treated but the practitioner or student should be able to introduce the modifications required by the patient's age, physical type and general health state.

Particular age groups need particular attention with regard to possible pathology of degeneration on the one hand to adaptation to the specific needs of children on the other.

Gross modifications to basic technique need to be considered where there are large anatomical variations. As an example a patient may have a fixed knee from an old osteomyelitis. This would make any technique requiring knee flexion impossible. This could be a nuisance but would not be insurmountable. However if a patient could not lie prone, for any reason, this could severely limit the range of techniques available, which would need some ingenuity from the operator. The ultimate problems occur in this area when called upon to work in a domiciliary situation, on the soft bed which is pushed up against a wall. The patient in this case is usually in acute pain, they are distressed and anxious, and they are often fixed in supine lying. This sort of situation can test to the limit the operator's skill in adapting treatment techniques!

APPLICATION OF CRANIAL TECHNIQUES

The techniques relating to cranial osteopathy are documented well in other works, and only the outline is discussed here for completeness.

Osteopathic technique does not stop at the atlas. Cranial osteopathy embraces the concept that there is mobility between the cranial bones. This movement is very small, but is measurable, and distortions in the movement patterns can be responsible for signs and symptoms locally and elsewhere. There are three broad approaches to the techniques designed to deal with these dysfunctions.

Firstly the cranial articular mechanism is considered. Secondly the membranous structures of the falx cerebelli, tentorium and meninges are amenable to technical approaches. The third aspect relates to the inherent motility of the cerebro-spinal fluid. As in all other techniques, the subdivisions are purely arbitrary and used primarily for recording and dialogue purposes.

The traditional teaching in this method uses the description "involuntary mechanism". The rhythmical oscillatory nature of this mechanism is palpable to the trained hand, and is amenable to alteration and variation with techniques designed specifically for this purpose. This is an exceptionally delicate method of treatment, and to the uninitiated, may seem totally bizarre. Nevertheless many manually dextrous osteopaths embrace this method as a supplement to, and sometimes as a complete replacement for, the more traditional methods. This fact alone makes the approach worthy of study. Why else, other than results, would a busy, successful practitioner choose to utilise any therapeutic method?

The rhythmic impulse can be palpated all over the body, not just at the head.

The simplest way to feel this is to sit in a relaxed position with the hand very lightly applied to the patient, with the operator's own elbow supported and acting as a pivot. The actual rhythmic impulse can be felt as a swelling and receding, or an ebbing and flowing. It sometimes takes some time to acquire the palpatory awareness necessary for this type of method. Very rarely will a practitioner have this skill at the outset, and the method therefore receives an undue amount of criticism from those unable or unwilling to acquire this skill.

When the patient's rhythm has been "tuned into", particularly if there is acute pain or distress, there will often be a considerable calming and relaxation. Sometimes there will be symptoms of heat, tingling, floating or lightness. This is not faith healing, as no faith is necessary to perceive this aspect of human energy, only a faith in the ability to believe what is being felt!

The rhythmic impulse of the involuntary mechanism is generally about 12 cycles per minute. The length of time before a practitioner can hope to become adept at palpating the rhythmic impulse and therefore start to use it in treatment varies greatly. This is of course true of many technical procedures, and it is necessary to have personal instruction in this method to be able to translate the palpatory findings into usable treatment techniques.

This facility can be gained by most people who are prepared to open their minds to the possibility of the concept. As with all other techniques, some patients are much more likely to benefit than others, and the selection as to which treatment should be applied and to which patient, remains part of the art of osteopathy.

This very brief outline is not in any way meant to be a full elaboration on cranial osteopathy or cranial techniques, but purely an item of information for those who have no knowledge whatsoever of the concept.

Some time spent practising the palpation of involuntary movements, preferably under supervision, is considered a useful method of improving any operator's palpatory awareness, even if there is no desire to go further and use these techniques as treatment procedures.

The one proviso which needs to be stated is that, if reactions are being induced, the palpation should be stopped.

Severe reactions, albeit temporary, are possible with injudicious cranial work. Palpation of the rhythmic impulse is better performed remote from the skull.

THE PHOTOGRAPHS

The photographs are organised in sequences to attempt to show (a) the position of the patient, (b) the hand position, where this needs to be clarified and (c) the position at the completion of the technique.

It may not be evident at first glance that there is any difference between the starting position and the final position. However a careful study of the pictures will show several subtle changes which are the very essence of the technique.

It is impossible to show every technique position but an attempt has been made to cover a representative sample for each area. Some of the positions will seem completely incomprehensible if the reader is not familiar with the particular technique, hence the availability from the publishers of a video tape of the techniques illustrated here being shown in action. Every one of these techniques, and many others, are tried and tested and have stood the test of time in that they are mostly classical osteopathic procedures.

The arrows are purely for guidance and give only rough guides as to the directions of movement but nevertheless give a useful starting point for development of the techniques. As has been said earlier, most techniques must be carried out in a curving plane to find the optimum direction for effectiveness.

Not all these techniques will be useful for all operators, due to differences in size, strength of thumbs, weight etc. Sufficient variations are shown to avoid this being a major problem.

Section A
Techniques for the cervical region

Kneading paravertebral muscles

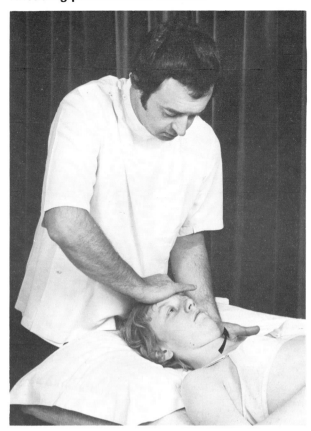

The operator's right hand is holding back on the forehead with an equal and opposite pressure as the left hand which is stretching and kneading the paravertebral muscles on the left, pulling them gently from the spinous processes laterally and waiting until a sense of relaxation is felt.

Kneading and articulation simultaneously

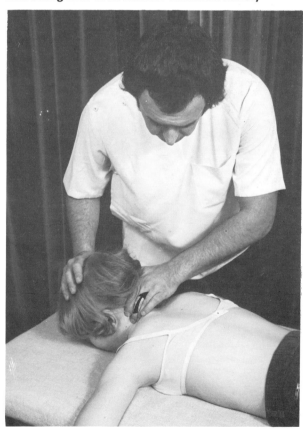

This soft tissue stretching technique is performed prone, which has the advantage that the operator's other hand can apply a rolling articulatory movement at the same time. The transverse processes are very sensitive and therefore care must be taken not to put undue pressure on them in this technique.

Kneading paravertebral muscles

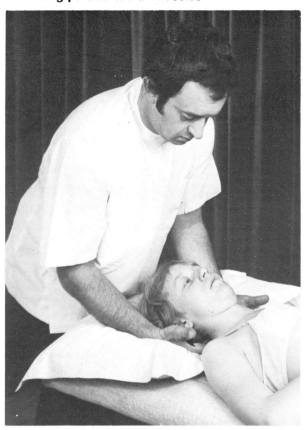

The hands are applied to the paravertebral muscles on both sides and the fingers flexed slowly to produce stretch. The palms are away from the head in this case so that the wrists can rest on the table, or pillow and form a fulcrum.

Kneading, stretching and articulation

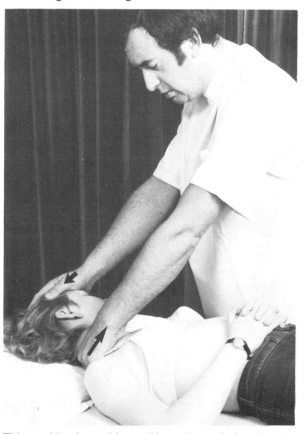

This combined stretching and kneading technique has the advantage that the operator need only lean back to increase the power, and the other hand can perform a variety of different movements combined with the stretch.

41

Strong articulation with kneading

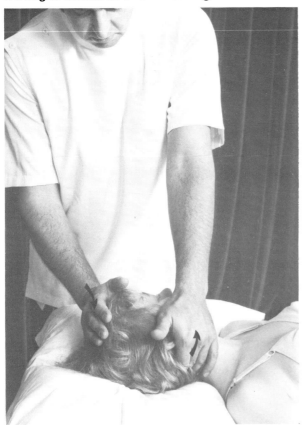

This alternative hold for combined soft tissue stretching and articulation is a variation which allows the operator to roll the head with the other hand and using a combination of side-bending and rotation to the other side, stabilise the spine and produce very strong stretching.

Stretch of scaleni using head

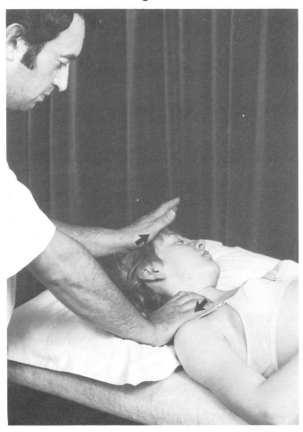

This hold allows the head to be rotated to the opposite side from the stretch, which in this case is away from the throat. There are times when this is a necessary direction.

Kneading and stretch of scaleni

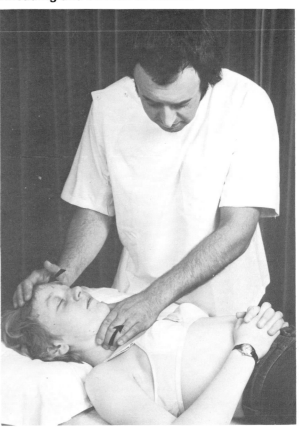

The anterior tissues of the neck can be reached with this hold. The scaleni and sternomastoid can be worked, whilst the head is being gently rolled in the opposite direction.

Kneading of anterior neck muscles

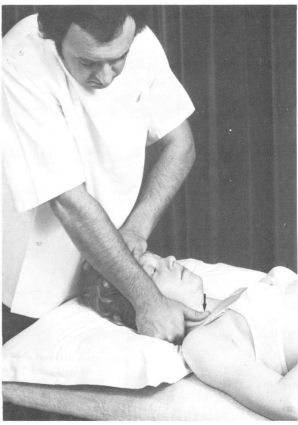

This approach to the anterior tissues of the neck is useful as the muscles can be stretched away from the throat while the head is being rolled simultaneously in either direction. Alternatively the muscles can be held on a constant stretch and the head rolling acts as the stretching force.

Hand position for occipital springing

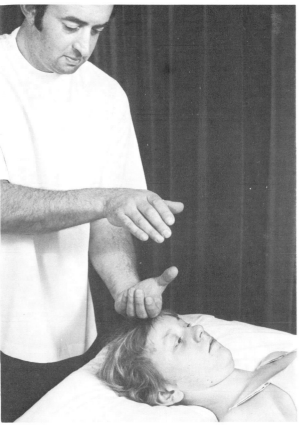

This shows the basic position of the hands for the hold used in occipital springing.

Occipital springing

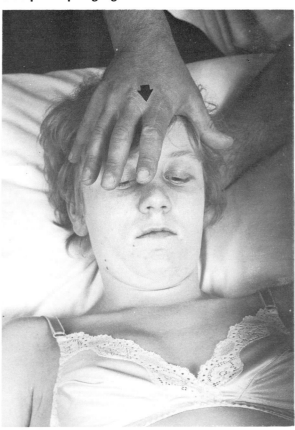

The hands are applied with the patient's forehead and the atlanto-occipital area as the contact points.

Occipital springing in extension

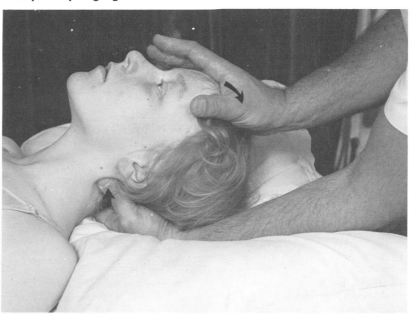

This shows how the basic hold can be used to produce a localised extension of the occiput.

43

Occipital springing with traction

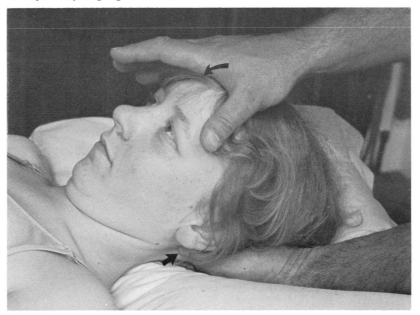

This shows how, using the same hold as the extension leverage, flexion can be achieved at the atlanto-occipital junction.

Occipital springing

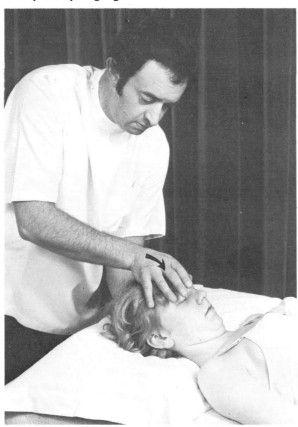

The operator's posture is shown here to emphasise the use of body weight and an upright position rather than the use of arm power.

Hold for universal movements in occipital springing

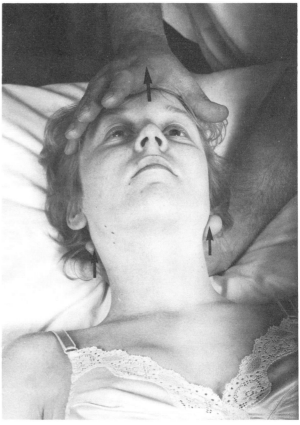

The operator's fingers are spread over a wider area in this hold to reduce the pressure on the posterior tissues which may be very tender. This hold also allows the movements of side-bending and rotation without changing hand positions.

Occipital springing in flexion/side-bending

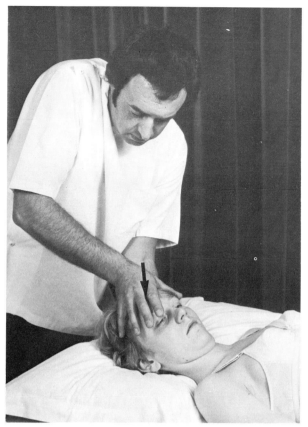

Using the same basic hold the occiput can be side-bent in flexion by a small variation in hand direction.

Occipital springing in extension/side-bending

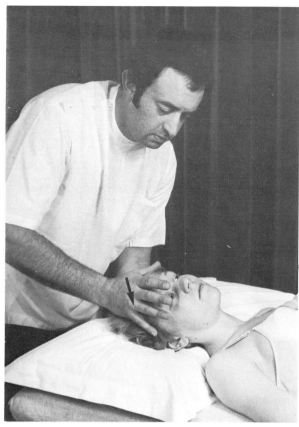

This shows another variation, namely side-bending in extension.

Stretching lateral neck tissues

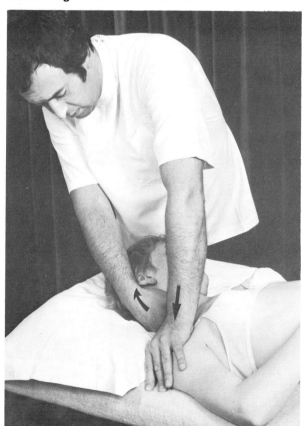

The right hand in this case is placed with the fingers fixing round the spinous processes and the head is pulled progressively into side-bending and rotation while the left hand helps localise the movement by counter-fixing on the shoulder. With small variations this can be modified into a technique using traction, and by varying the angle of counter-fixation against the shoulder, the force can be localised in different parts of the neck.

Stretching posterior neck tissues

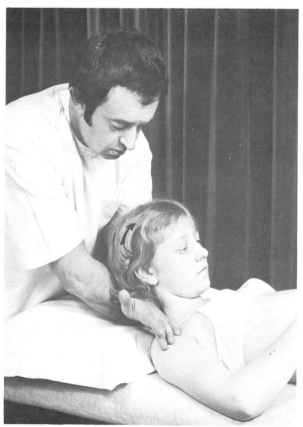

In this technique the patient's head is carefully balanced on the operator's crossed-wrists and with small variations in direction of force different parts of the neck can be stretched specifically.

Postero-lateral neck stretching

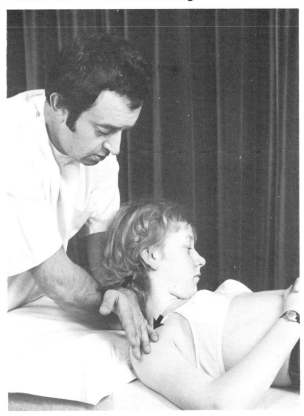

This shows the sort of variation possible with the cross-handed hold.

Cross-fibre kneading of trapezius

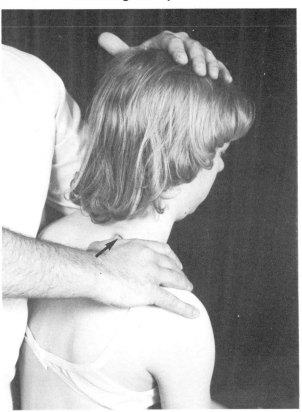

This position for cross-fibre kneading of trapezius was chosen to illustrate the use of the operator's body to support the patient. Also note the use of the other hand to stabilise the head. This could also be used to side-bend the neck to the right, to take the muscle off stretch, or to the left to increase the stretch. Rotation, flexion or extension could also be introduced if it was considered necessary.

Cross-fibre stretching of trapezius

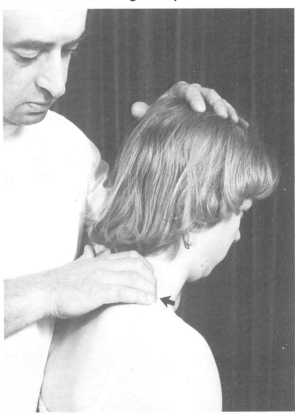

With only a small variation from the last hold shown, the technique can be varied to use the fingers instead of the thumb. In this case the technique of soft-tissue stretching could be extended to the scaleni muscles as well as trapezius.

Occipital articulation in extension

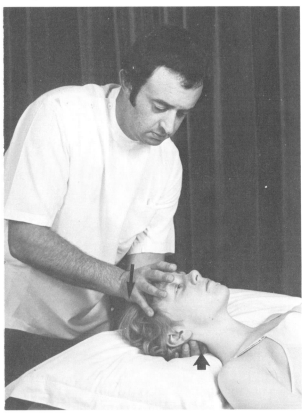

This variation of the occipital articulation methods shows extension, using the operator's underneath hand as a fulcrum. This can be combined with side-bending and rotation if desired.

Upper cervical side-bending

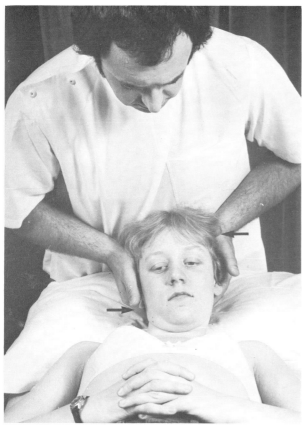

This hold allows side-bending to be performed at the upper cervical area. Note that the operator's hands are staggered so that the fingers of the right hand can form a fulcrum. The head is in flexion in this case and the vertex is pressed into the operator's abdomen. Extension could just as easily be induced.

Upper cervical side-bending with rotation

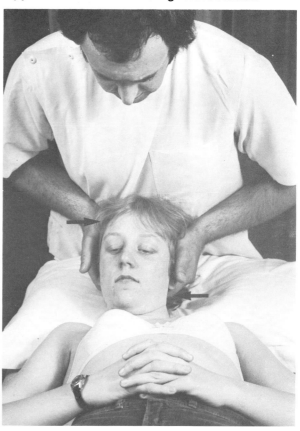

This hold is similar to the previous one except that a small degree of rotation has been induced to the opposite side to the side-bending to help localise the force to a more specific point.

Mid cervical side-bending

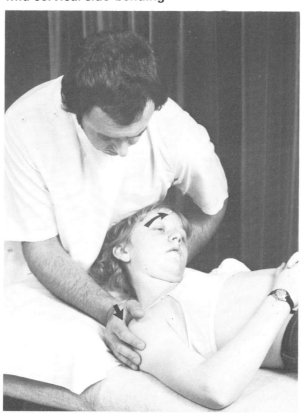

In this hold the head is being side-bent and rotated to the right as the shoulder is firmly pushed down to stretch the lateral cervical muscles. Varying degrees of rotation and flexion can be used to direct the force to specific areas in the neck. Note that the operator's chest is being used to assist the leverage.

Traction with side-bending

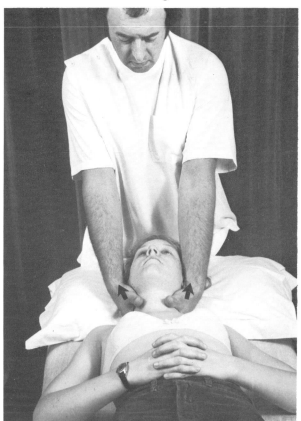

Traction with side-bending

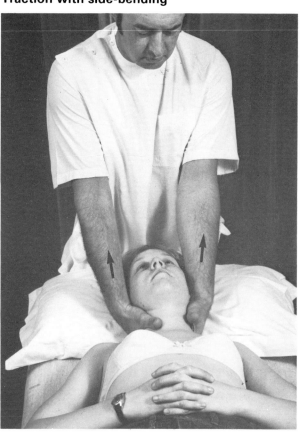

In these two pictures the neck is being put on traction at the same time as side-bending is being introduced alternately to either side. The traction is induced with the thenar eminences under the mandible, the hypothenar eminences under the occiput and the thumbs gently applied under the mandible. The side-bending is induced by the operator rotating his own spine and pressing alternately on the transverse processes on either side.

Postero-anterior springing

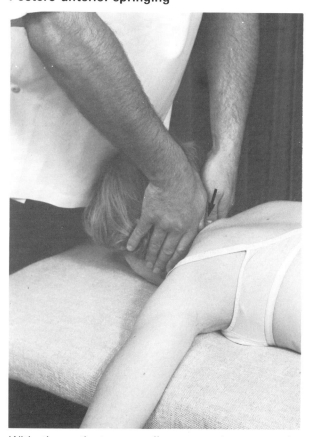

With the patient prone direct posterior to anterior springing can be applied over the lateral masses of the cervical vertebrae. If this is performed over the spinous processes it is likely to be painful and care must be taken to avoid this.

Side-shifting springing

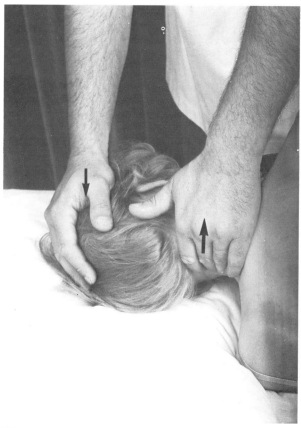

With the patient side-lying, the operator's right hand is stabilising the head and the other hand is pulling gently so that the neck is side-bent. This technique also is very useful as a diagnostic procedure to localise areas of restricted flexibility which will be readily palpable due to the restricted side-shifting possible.

Extension and rotation springing

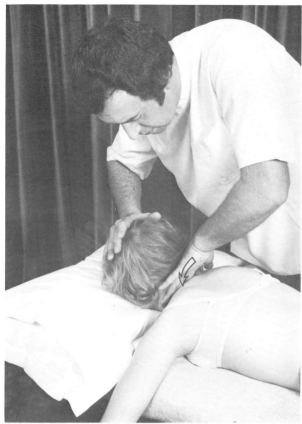

The neck is placed in extension here and the operator is pushing on the posterior of the transverse processes on the patient's left side. This produces a very localised extension and rotation. Using side-bending to the opposite side to the rotation force, this procedure can be transformed into a thrust procedure, although it is difficult to control the amplitude with the patient prone.

Localised side-bending

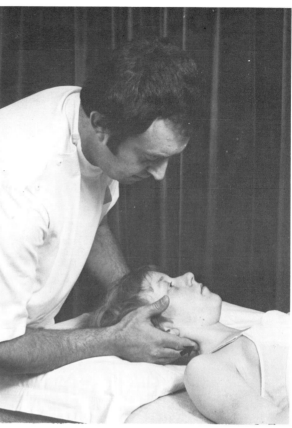

This hold can be a follow on from the usual position for soft-tissue techniques and localised side-bending, with different degrees of the other possible ranges, can be induced.

Localised side-bending and side-shifting

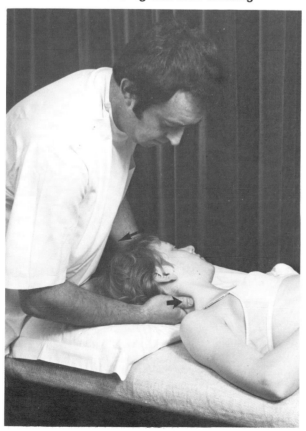

The operator's thumb is the fulcrum to induce side-bending, and localise the force whilst the other hand alters the head position to optimise the tension produced.

Localised rotatation

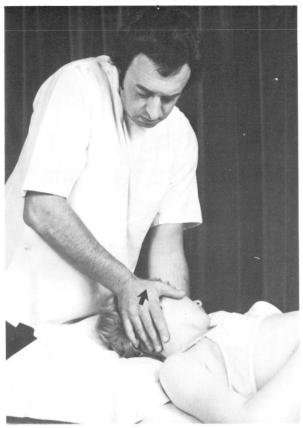

The right hand is producing rotation whilst the left, in this case is holding back on the transverse processes on the patient's left side to induce a localised rotation in the upper cervical area.

Localised flexion

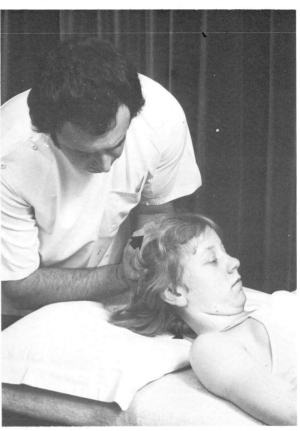

The patient's head is being gently pushed into flexion whilst the operator's other hand is back on the spinous processes to produce a fixation point.

Minimal leverage thrust for atlas

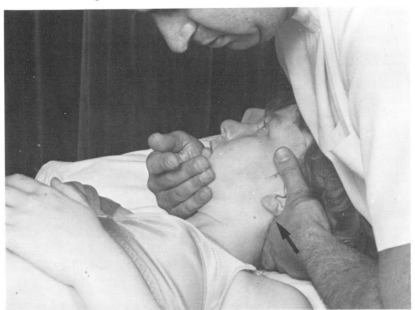

This shows the position for the application of a minimal leverage thrust technique as applied to the posterior arch of the atlas. Note that the patient's head is not in full rotation, neither is it in full side-bending or in fact in any leverage position. It is placed so that the contact point is available to the applicator, in this case slight rotation, slight extension, and very slight side-bending to the left. The neck is gently moved around until full relaxation is felt. The actual thrust in this case is applied as a very rapid contraction of the operator's brachioradialis and pectorals whilst holding the head firmly with the other hand to prevent any further movement occurring. At the culmination of the thrust, using this category of technique the neck never reaches a full leverage position.

Combined leverage and thrust for atlas

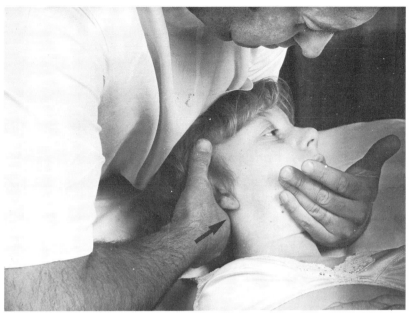

This technique is a combined leverage and thrust approach. The head is gently rotated to the left and then side-bent and extended only just sufficiently to make the soft tissues over the arch of the atlas relaxed so that the thrusting hand can be pressed firmly but gently in under the occiput. The angle of thrust in this case is upwards towards the left eye of the patient. The operator's left hand does not pull the chin around, it merely stabilises the head. This type of technique can be made into a momentum approach by slowly oscillating back and forth until the optimum tension is sensed under the thrusting hand.

Combined leverage and thrust to atlas with traction

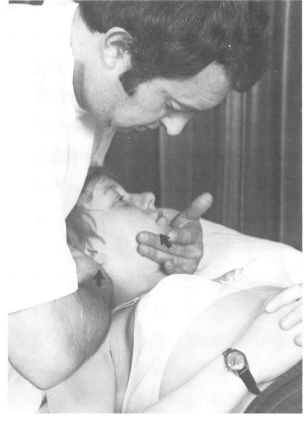

This shows a traction modification of the combined leverage method where the operator uses both hands to produce a firm traction at the moment of thrust. If there are degenerative changes in the lower cervical spine this modification will enable the upper cervical area to be treated without stressing the lower neck excessively. In the presence of degenerative changes of any consequence. ALL cervical thrust techniques should be carefully controlled.

Combined leverage and thrust in traction and side-bending

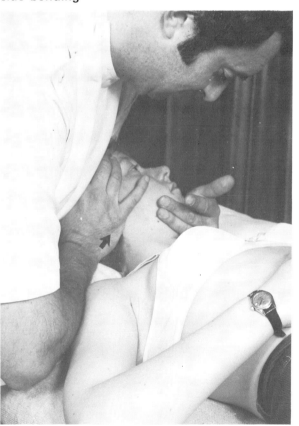

This shows an alternative hold for the traction type of thrust. This has the advantage that side-bending forces to gap the opposite side can be introduced relatively easily.

51

Atlas thrust in side-bending

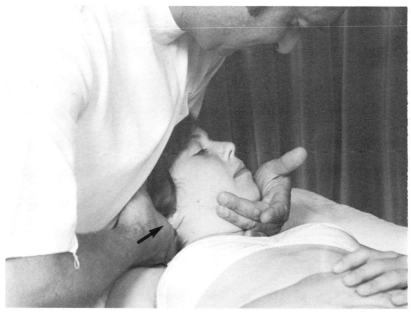

The hold shown here is for a pure side-bending thrust as applied to the atlas.

Gapping thrust for left occipito-atlantal joint

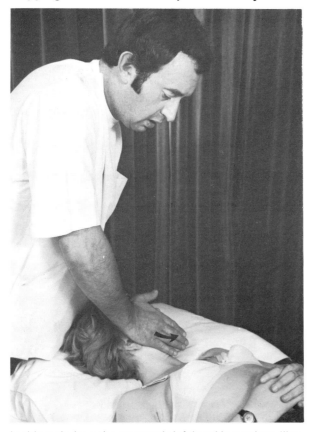

In this technique the operator's left hand is gently pulling up on the patient's left occiput and the right hand is pushing on the maxilla and the mandible into extension, side-bending and rotation. The tension is occurring in the atlanto-occipital joint nearest the table.

Thrust directed to right occipito-atlantal joint

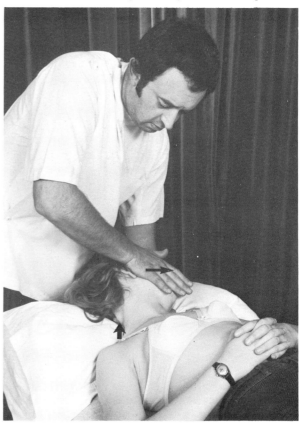

This hold utilises rotation and side-bending to the same side, pivoting over the operator's left hand which is pushing up to the ceiling. The right hand is maintaining the side-bending and then thrusting on the maxilla into rotation to open the patient's right occipito-atlantal joint and drive the occiput forwards.

Hold for atlas 'tug' (1)

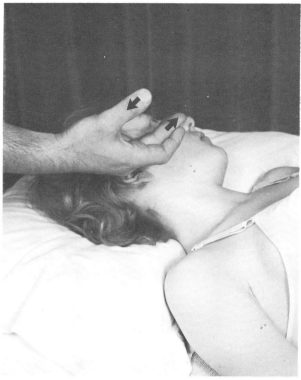

This technique uses the principle of contra-rotation in an unusual way. The operator's right hand is going to pull the atlas into rotation to the right despite the fact that the neck is rotated to the left. The fingers will push up on the arch of the atlas on the other side and the thumb will be held gently over the transverse process of the atlas to pull it backwards on that side at the completion of the procedure.

Hold applied (2)

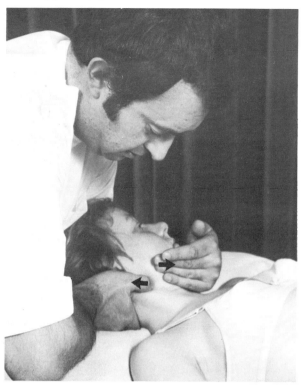

The operator's left hand is now applied to the mandible and gently oscillates the head into rotation to the left a few times, whilst at the same time pulling the atlas into rotation to the right.

Atlas 'tug' completed (3)

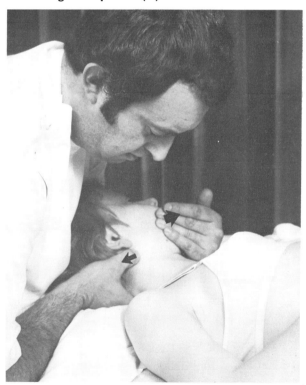

At the completion of the technique note that the operator's right elbow has dropped closer to the table. The left hand has rotated the head further to the left at the same time. The head does not in fact have to reach full rotation and the atlas pressure is firm but only applied momentarily to avoid undue discomfort. This technique, although difficult to perform well, is very useful as it is possible to introduce contra-rotation without extreme movement, and without rotating the head towards the side on which one is trying to produce gapping.

Prone combined leverage and thrust to atlas

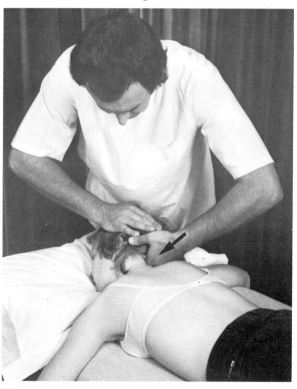

Using the basic principles of side-bending to one side with rotation to the other, with the added use of either flexion or extension, the prone position is available for thrust techniques. In this position it is imperative that there is no follow through in the thrust, to avoid the possibility of over-extending the neck. If suitable care is taken, this position can be very effective.

53

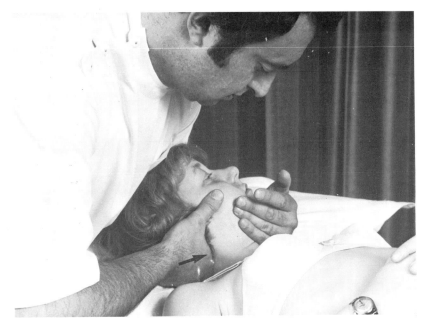

Side-bending combined leverage and thrust applied to gap left facet (1)

The direction of thrust can control the effective action of this technique. In this case the thrusting hand is directed towards the patient's left shoulder.

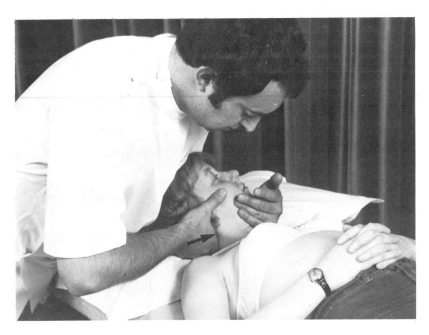

Completion of thrust (2)

This shows the completion of the technique. The operator's left forearm has produced a slight accentuation of side-bending over the fulcrum of the right hand. Note that the thrusting forearm has remained horizontal throughout.

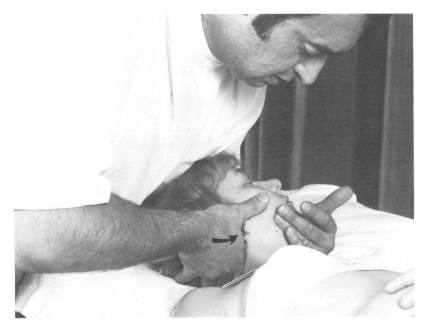

Rotation combined leverage and thrust

The chin hold combined leverage and thrust is being used here as a rotation thrust, the direction being towards the patient's left eye. The left hand acts purely as a stabiliser, it does not pull on the chin. The operator's wrist is allowed to fall into ulnar flexion and then is accelerated through a very small range to rotate the neck.

Cradle hold for cervical thrusts

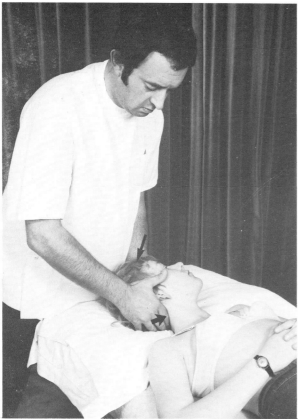

This cradle hold is a very useful variation from the usual chin hold which many operators find cumbersome, and many patients find uncomfortable. The operator's interphalangeal joint is pushed firmly into the soft tissues behind the transverse processes and the other hand is cupping the other side of the head. The thrust is performed as a combination of a rapid pronation of the operator's right hand and a similar supination of his left.

Sitting combined leverage and thrust hold (1)

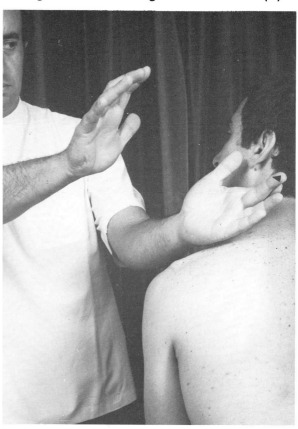

Localised articulation and thrust techniques can be performed with the patient in a sitting position. The hand positions and applicator are shown here.

Sitting thrust applied behind transverse process (2)

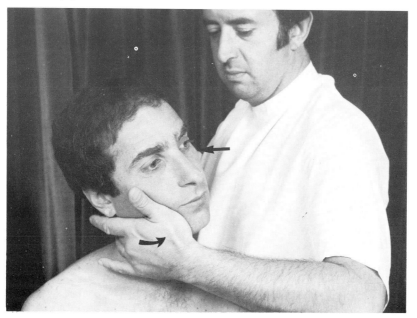

The hands are applied and the operator's left hand is firmly contacting the mandible and the posterior aspect of the transverse processes. The right hand is putting equal and opposite pressure on the other side of the head.

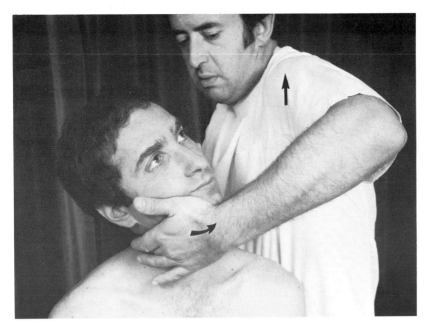

Lower cervical sitting rotation and traction thrust

This shows the after thrust position. Note the operator's thrusting hand has pulled the neck further into rotation in the rotation direction, and that the vertex has been taken slightly off the mid line.

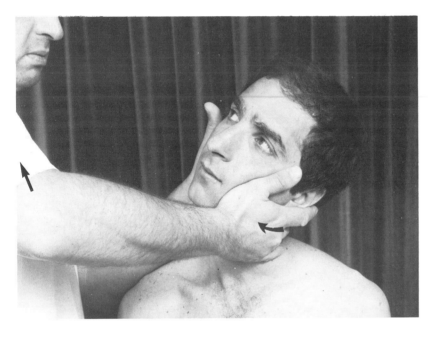

Upper cervical sitting rotation thrust (1)

This shows the same rotation technique, performed this time as applied to the C2-3 joint. The difference between this direction and the previous one is that more rotation is being used, which is more effective in the upper cervical area.

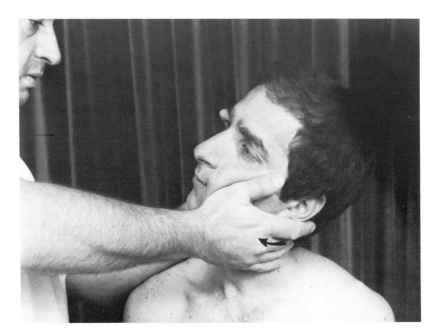

Upper cervical sitting rotation thrust completed (2)

This shows the after thrust position. Note the horizontal position of the forearm.

Mid cervical side-bending thrust (1)

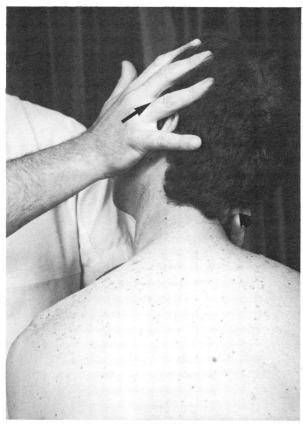

This shows the side-bending approach from behind.

Mid cervical side-bending thrust completed (2)

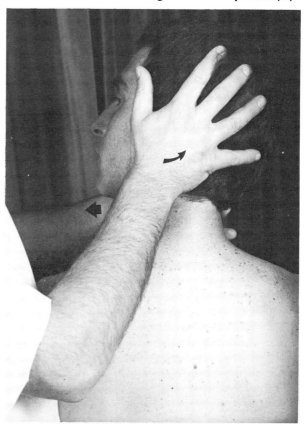

This shows the after thrust position, note the head hand is covering the ear and has pushed the head into side-bending at the same time as the other hand pulled on the transverse processes.

Occipito-atlantal thrust (1)

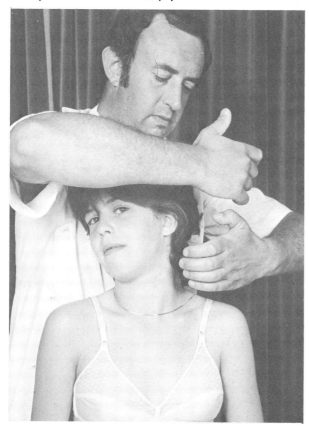

The basic position for applying a thrust to the occipito-atlantal joint in a sitting position, where the operator can hold back on the atlas, and pull the occiput forward is shown here.

Occipito-atlantal thrust hold applied (2)

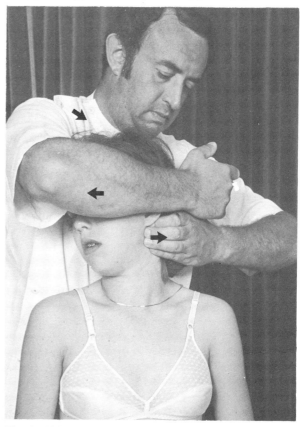

The hold is applied here. The operator is comfortably holding on the anterior surface of the transverse process of the atlas. The other forearm is pressing the head into rotation, and pushing it into the operator's own chest with pressure on the parietal area. This will cause the head to be side-bent away from the operator as the technique is completed.

Occipito-atlantal thrust completed (3)

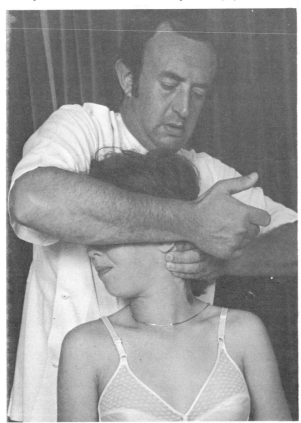

Here the technique is completed. The operator has firmly, but only momentarily held back on the transverse process of the atlas. He has abducted his right arm at the same time as pushing it in towards himself. This produces rotation of the occiput to the right and of the atlas to the left. At the same time the head is side-bent to the left to allow slack in the joint to aid gapping. Because the technique is performed between the two hands, rather than at the extreme of movement, it can be performed without using full rotation, which might be undesirable for a variety of reasons.

Traction in side-bending

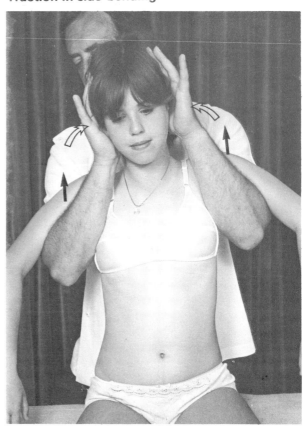

This hold is useful if traction and side-bending is needed in the cervical spine. Some of the patient's weight is taken via the shoulders, and the thenar eminences of the operator are locked under the mastoid processes to direct the force to the neck.

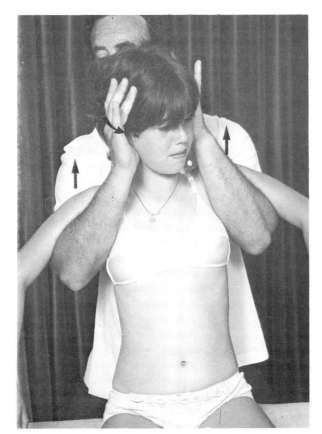

Traction in rotation

A similar hold to that used in the last technique is shown here, the main difference being that rotation is being induced with traction rather than any other movement. Naturally, all movement directions can be brought into play as necessary.

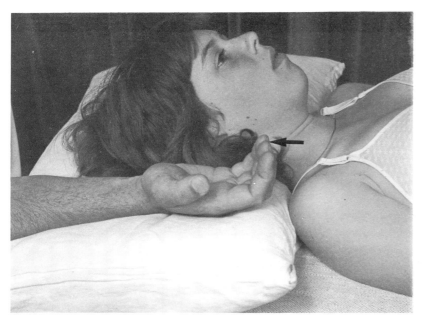

Specific upper cervical traction (1)

The hand is shown apart from the head here to show the finger position used to apply specific traction to the upper cervical spine.

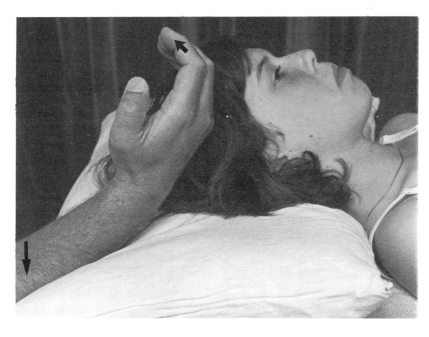

Specific upper cervical traction (2)

If the previous hold is applied under the occiput, and then the forearm is pivoted over the end of the table, strong traction can be used with very little effort.

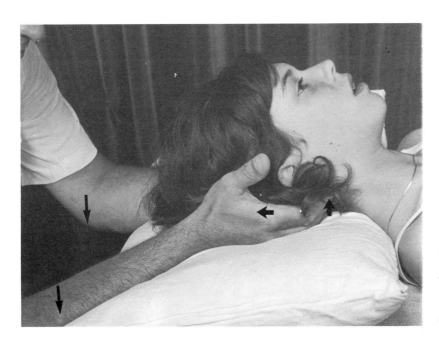

Specific upper cervical traction (3)

The complete technique hold is shown here. Note that very little effort is necessary to produce quite strong traction when using this hold.

Section B
Techniques for the thoracic region and ribs

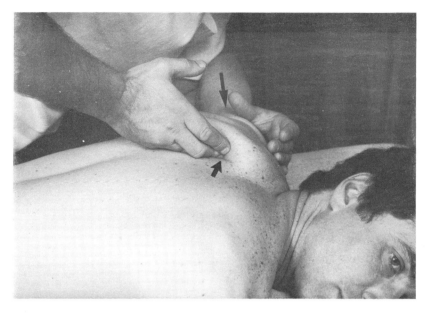

Kneading inter-scapular muscles

The muscles under, and medial to the scapula can be reached with this technique. The operator's left hand is pushing the scapula medially to enable the other hand to get under the scapula.

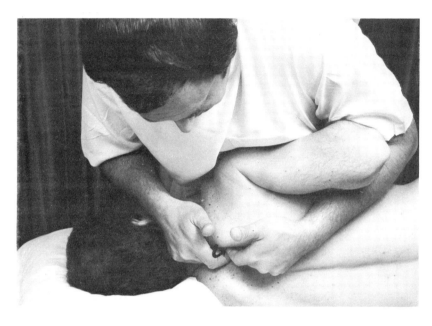

Kneading inter-scapular muscles

The scapular muscles are accessible in the side-lying position with this technique. The operator's body is applying pressure to the shoulder and the fingers can then be worked under the scapula.

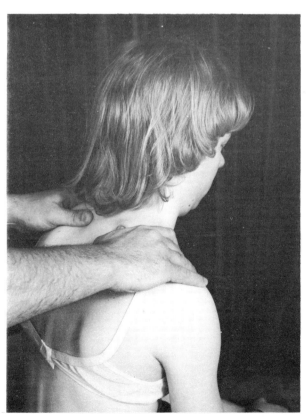

Sitting kneading to trapezius

This shows one of the most comfortable holds for applying soft-tissue cross-fibre kneading to the horizontal fibres of trapezius.

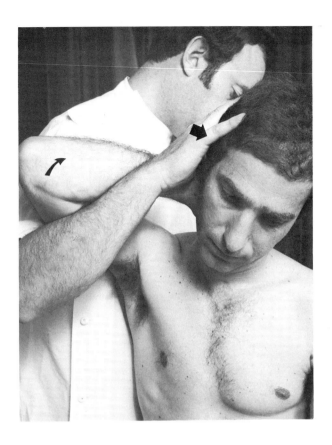

Reinforced side-bending cervico-dorsal area

Very strong side-bending can be applied to the cervico-dorsal region with this hold. It can be reinforced with the operator applying his free thumb to the concavity formed in the C/D area to localise the forces. Even stronger side-bending, and therefore foraminal gapping can be used if the operator extends the patient's shoulder at the same time as applying the side-bending force.

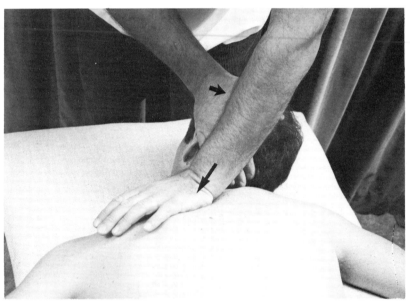

Prone cervico-dorsal thrust

The upper thoracic area can be manipulated in many positions. The hold shown here is used when the operator wishes to gap the apophyseal joints on the left. The applicator can be applied to several different contact points. In this case the transverse processes are being used. The head is slowly rotated to the left as the right side-bending is maintained. As tension is sensed at the operator's left hypothenar eminence, a short thrust is applied towards the patient's left axilla. If the rib angle was being thrust, the direction would be towards the pelvis. If the spinous process was being thrust the direction would be towards the patient's left shoulder.

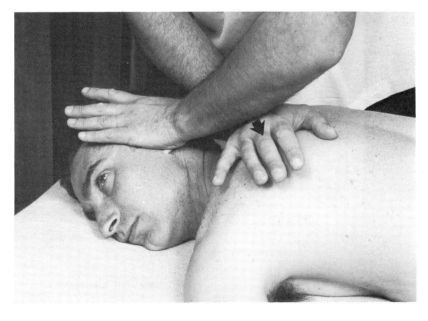

Prone cervico-dorsal thrust (crossed hands)

This alternative hold for applying thrust techniques to the upper thoracic area is more suitable for some operators. The position of the patient has not altered from the previous technique, but the hand position has. Note that the hand applied to the head is above the thrusting hand, this ensures that the neck is not wrenched excessively when the thrust is applied.

Prone cervico-dorsal thrust using pisiform

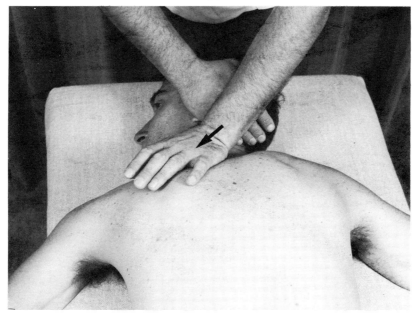

Here there is another variation of holds for the same basic technique. In this case the operator has placed the head in a greater degree of rotation and therefore there is less side-bending available. The head hand is primarily a stabiliser, it does not thrust, merely holds back whilst the other hand performs the main part of the technique.

Prone cervico-dorsal thrust using thumb (1)

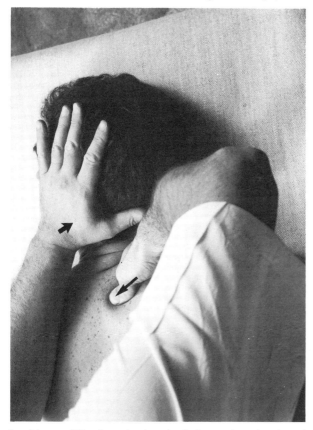

In this modification the head of the patient is placed exactly as in the previous technique. The operator has moved from the end of the table to stand at the patient's side (either side according to preference). The head hand is once again a stabiliser, and the thrust comes from the operator's thumb applied to the lamina of the vertebra. It is pushed gently forwards then towards the patient's axilla. Note that the operator's forearm is in line with the thumb.

Prone cervico-dorsal thrust using thumb (2)

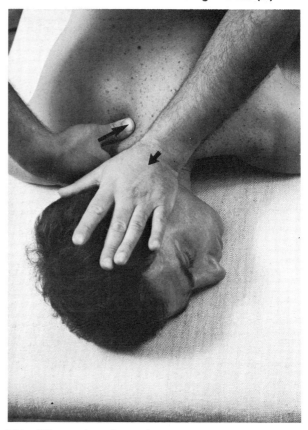

This different view shows the operator inducing a greater degree of rotation and traction than the previous picture. Note that the head is not side-bent out of the mid line.

Prone cervico-dorsal springing/thrust

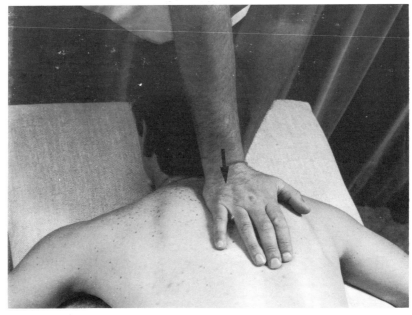

This strong technique can be applied to patients whose necks are capable of full extension without excessive discomfort. The operator is pulling gently on the chin and applying a counter-force on the spinous processes in an oscillating manner. The thrust is applied with very low amplitude at the point of optimum tension, towards the patient's sternum.

Sitting cervico-dorsal thrust (1)

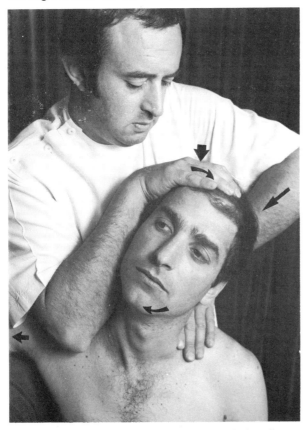

The basic positions of leverage utilising side-bending to one side and rotation to the other are used in this technique. The operator's right hand is producing side-bending, reverse rotation and some compression. The left thumb is applied to the spinous process of the segment being worked and the thrust is towards the patient's right axilla. In this particular case the operator has placed the patient's arm over his thigh to impart greater stability and assist the side-bending forces as well.

Sitting cervico-dorsal thrust (2)

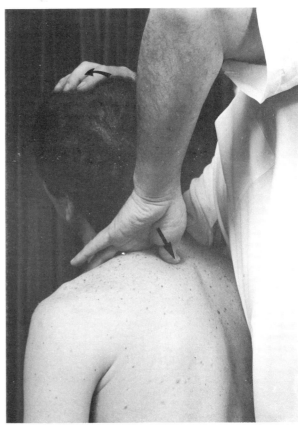

This shows the same technique as the previous picture but the rear view is used to demonstrate the thumb position for the thrust.

Sitting cervico-dorsal thrust using pisiform

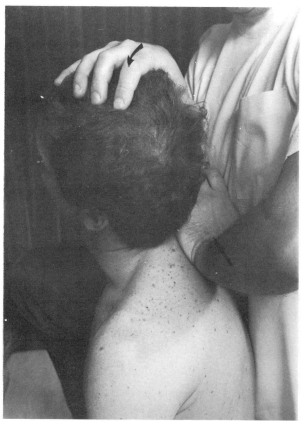

This side-on view shows a further modification in the same technique using the hypothenar eminence instead of the thumb. This is useful for operators who find that thumb strength is inadequate.

Side-lying cervico-dorsal thrust head hold

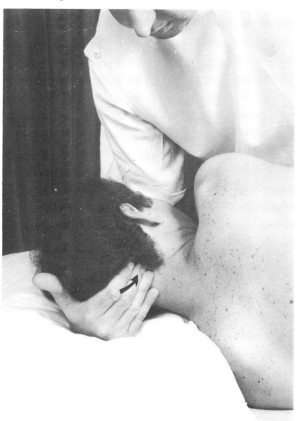

The basic position for a side-lying approach to the upper thoracic area is shown here. Note the operator's right hand is placed in such a way that full control of the head is maintained.

Side-lying cervico-dorsal thrust hand position

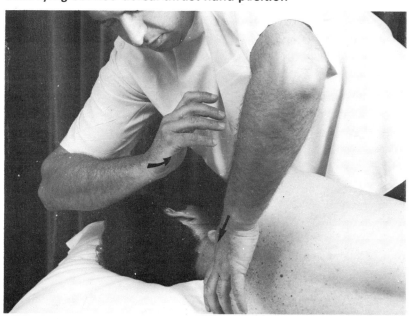

The hands are shown here in the position they will assume at the completion of the thrust.

Side-lying cervico-dorsal thrust basic position

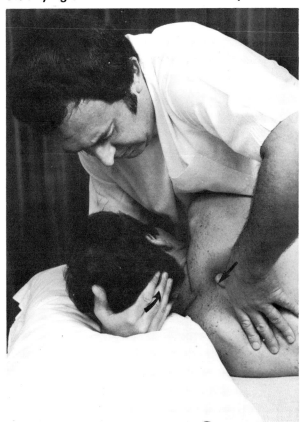

The hands here are applied, although no leverages have been developed. Note that the operator's chest is applied to the shoulder girdle to aid stability and induce some preliminary compression. The thrusting thumb is lightly applied at this stage to avoid undue discomfort.

Side-lying cervico-dorsal thrust final position

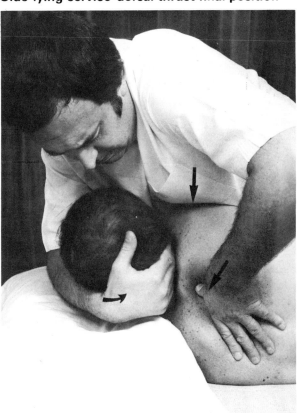

The final position after thrust demonstrates the reverse rotation of the head, the slight emphasis on side-bending and the primary emphasis on the thrust with the thumb. Note also the compression element with the operator's chest.

2nd alternative C/D thrust hold

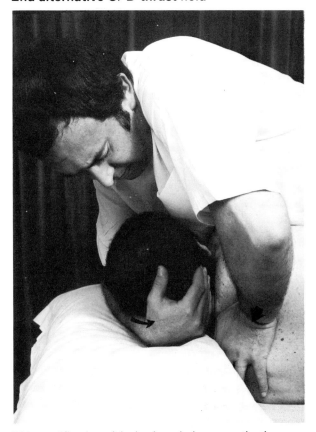

This modification of the basic technique uses the thenar or hypothenar eminence for the thrust if the thumb pressure is either too uncomfortable for the patient or the operator.

Alternative C/D thrust hold

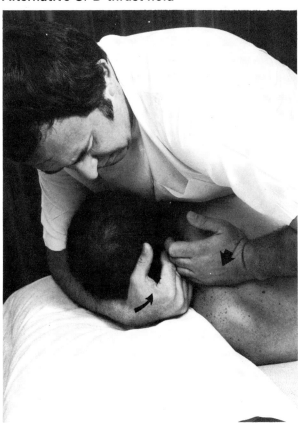

This further modification shows the operator using the hypothenar side of the hand for the thrust. It is difficult in this case to use the hand to perform a sharp enough thrust but if the patient's neck will take it, increased leverage can be applied to the head to achieve the same result.

Sitting dorsal (thoracic) articulation

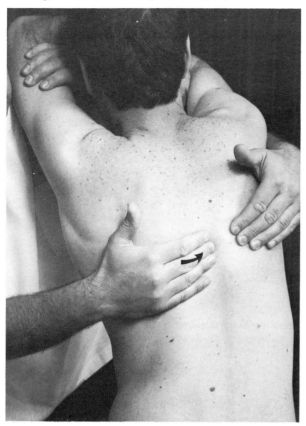

This sitting articulation position demonstrates a simple way of inducing side-bending and with it rotation to the same side, or the other side if desired to localise the forces to a specific point. This can be directed to the intervertebral joints, the costo-vertebral joints or the costotransverse joints.

Sitting dorsal and rib articulation

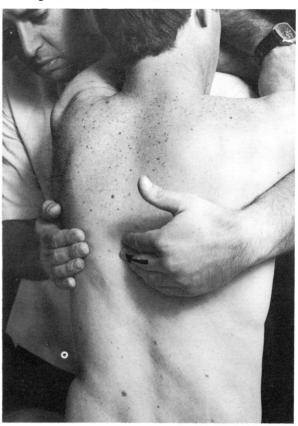

This alternative hold for articulating the dorsal column and ribs is sometimes more effective than the previous one in that the hands can both pull in the same direction whilst the shoulder girdle is tilted in the desired direction by the operator's own body position.

Sitting dorsal side-bending articulation

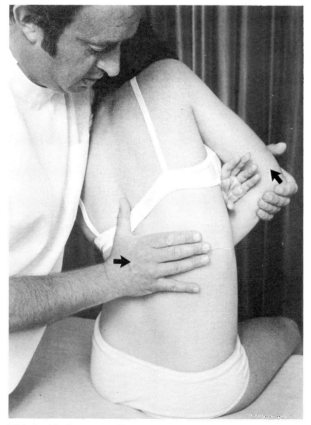

This hold allows an effective side-bending force in a fairly light subject. Either the thumb can be used as a fulcrum, or the thenar eminence.

Prone upper and mid-dorsal articulation

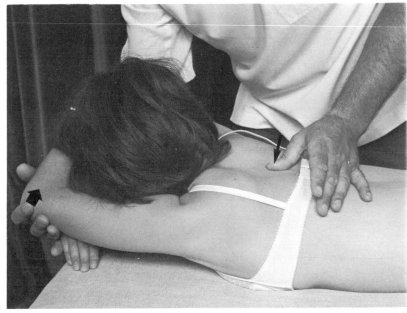

This hold is useful in a light subject to produce specific articulation from the upper, through to the mid to lower dorsal area. In this case side-bending is being introduced.

Sitting upper and mid-dorsal articulation

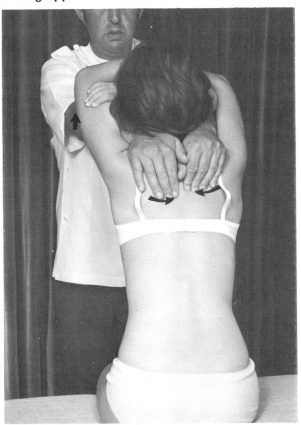

This hold is effective for mobilising the mid to upper dorsal area if the patient's shoulders are mobile enough to accept the position. Most directions of movement can be induced by subtle variations of force.

Side-lying rib articulation

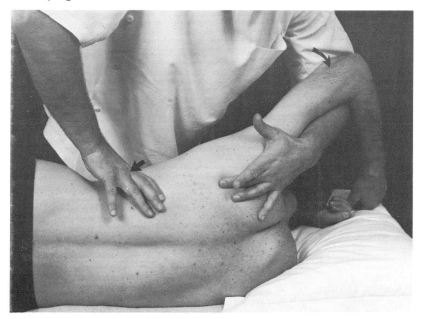

This side-lying position for rib articulation is made much more effective if the operator uses his cephalic hand to induce extension of the shoulder as well as elevation. At the same time the scapula is being firmly pressed against the chest wall so the leverage localises to the counter-fixing hand. The widest spread possible should be used with the hand on the ribs to minimise discomfort.

Supine rib articulation

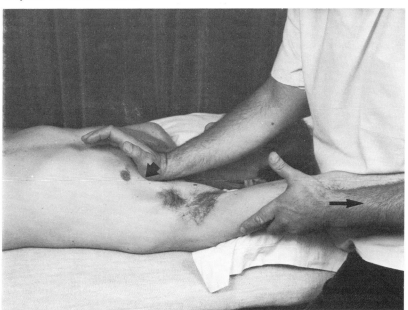

This supine technique for rib stretching uses the pull of the pectoral muscles counter-fixed with the operator's hand holding back on the lower of the two ribs which are to be spread. The patient's shoulder must be healthy, and different degrees of rotation of the shoulder can increase the effectiveness of the technique. Any technique designed to work on the ribs can be made more specific by using particular phases of respiration.

Supine rib articulation using thumb

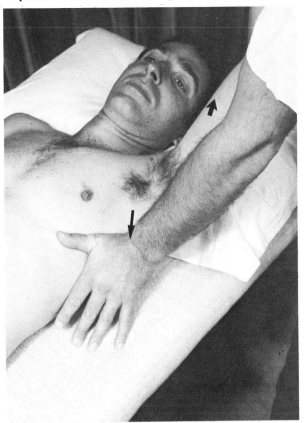

The operator's right hand here is elevating and flexing the shoulder whilst the fixing hand is holding back on the rib. Rotation of the patient's head to either side will also vary the effect of the technique.

Supine rib articulation using fingertips

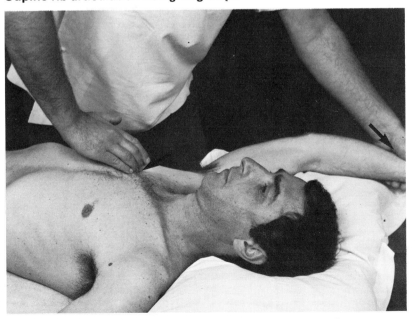

In this hold the operator is standing to the side of the patient instead of at the head. The fingertips are doing the fixing in this case.

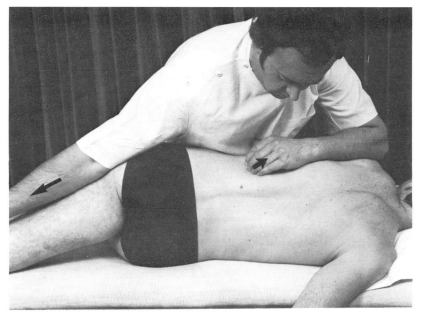

Side-lying lower rib articulation

This position is effective for articulating the lower ribs. The patient's upper leg is pushed into adduction and traction. The position of the spine in rotation tends to lock the vertebral component of movement and make the force much more effective at the costo-vertebral joints.

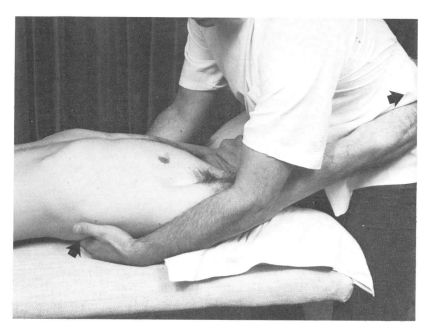

Supine dorsal and rib articulation in traction

In this technique traction is applied by the operator leaning back whilst the patient has clasped his hands around the operator's back. If the patient cannot reach, a towel or small pillow can be clasped between the hands to bridge the gap. The operator is prising up on the angles of the ribs, and rotation or side-bending can be induced by small changes in operator position. If the patient crosses one leg to the other this will also vary the localising of forces.

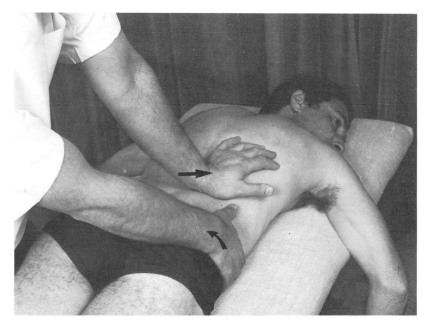

Prone dorso-lumbar and rib articulation

This articulatory technique for the lower ribs can be modified into a thrust technique in suitable cases. The operator's straight left arm is fixing on the rib angles with the hypothenar eminence. The right hand is pulling back on the anterior superior iliac spine. Before the pull back into rotation, the hand is pulled towards the operator. This induces a degree of compression which will minimise the amount of rotation necessary by the combination of compression and a small degree of side-bending. Variations in head rotation of the patient's head should be tried as this will affect the technique also.

73

Sitting rib thrust (1)

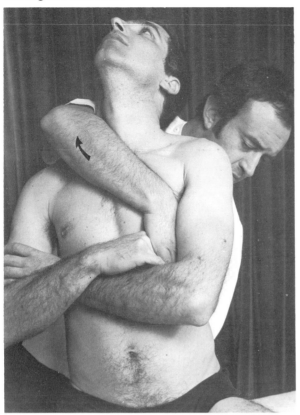

This technique is a very complex combination of leverages which is unusual in that the order of application of leverage alters the effectiveness and the comfort of the technique. Compression is applied by the operator pulling the chest-holding hand towards him. Side-bending to the right is applied, then rotation to the right and finally side-bending to the left at the same time as the extension force is applied to the angle of the rib with the other hand. The patient is asked to drop his head back into extension which assists the extension movement desired at the thrust point. If the side-bending and reverse rotation is applied at the same time it will be found that the spine locks up too quickly and the technique will not be effective. The production of the side-bending to the opposite side to the rotation at the last moment is usually more efficient. Several alternative holds can be applied if the chest hold is undesirable or impossible.

Sitting rib thrust (2)

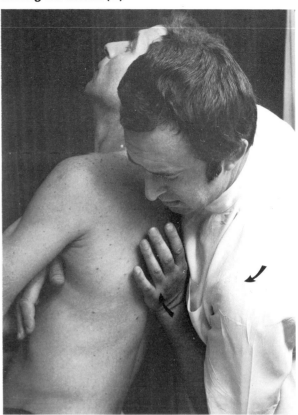

This shows the same technique as in the previous picture. The side view is shown of the thrust position. Note that the thrusting hand is nearly vertical, and that the thrusting arm is held close to the operator's side to increase the stability.

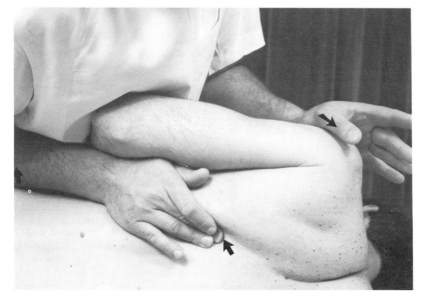

Side-lying rib articulation/thrust

Although the patient is in this case in a classical lumbar side-lying thrust position, the operator has applied a compression force to the pelvis and lower ribs and the force has been driven up towards the middle ribs. This can be made a very effective specific articulation or even into a thrust technique in suitable cases. This means of localising requires the operator to be careful not to stress the lumbar articulations excessively. If the prime part of the lower lever is compression not rotation, this will not be a problem.

Dorsal soft-tissue kneading

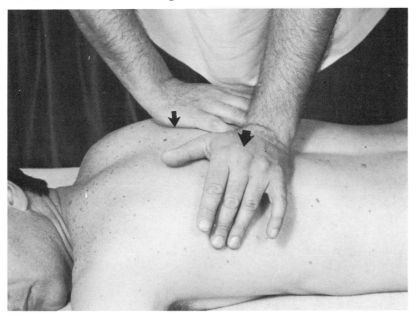

This picture shows a typical prone approach to applying soft-tissue kneading to the dorsal erector spinae muscles. Note the right hand is applying a downward force to stabilise the spine and prevent the kneading effect from producing too much rotation. Care is taken to avoid excessive skin stretch, by taking some slack in the skin before pushing the muscle bulk away from the spine.

Dorsal soft-tissue kneading

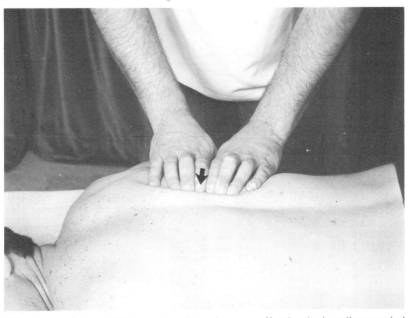

This approach to soft-tissue stretching is more effective in heavily muscled individuals. The paravertebral muscles are being pushed towards the spine with the fingertips. A wide spread of several fingertips avoids excessive discomfort.

Movement testing

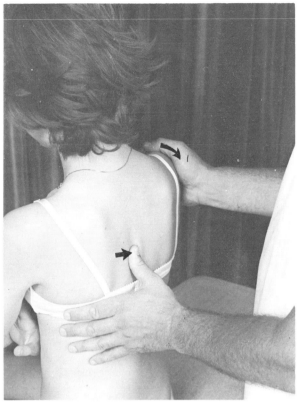

This very simple hold can be used for movement testing throughout the spine. It is most useful in the dorsal area. The operator's right hand is moving the patient's shoulder backwards and forwards through a small arc. At the same time the left hand is pressing lightly against the spinous processes one at a time. If this movement is performed fairly quickly, through a small range, a good idea of relative flexibility can be achieved. This will direct the operator to areas of significance.

Hold for dorsal articulation

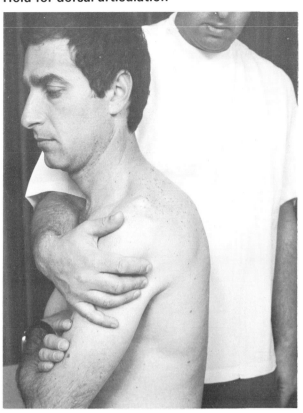

The dorsal spine can be mobilised using many holds. This basic position is useful as full control can be maintained whilst increased power can be induced by the addition of compression by the operator squeezing the patient's shoulders together.

Hold for dorsal articulation

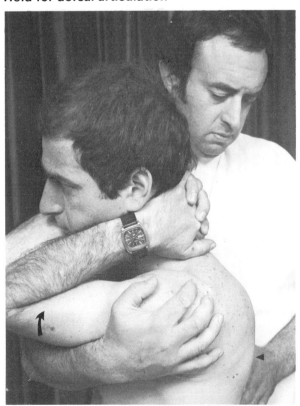

This hold allows very good control by the operator of the patient and various directions of force can be introduced. In this case extension is being performed. The operator is squeezing the patient's shoulders in towards his chest to stabilise the levers.

Hold for dorsal articulation

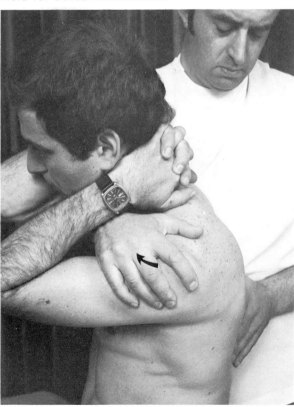

This alternative hold is useful if side-bending is required in combination with the rotation etc. The operator moves with the patient and thereby increases the effect of the technique.

Side-bending articulation using thumb

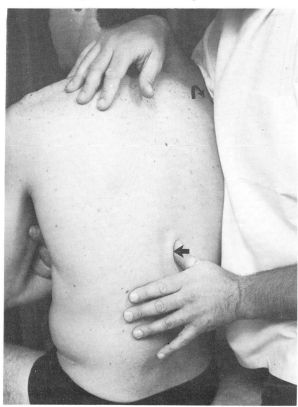

This simple hold for introducing side-bending can be used particularly when the patient is heavily built as little stress occurs on the operator and the thumb forms a useful fulcrum. The head must be kept above the pelvis to maintain stability.

Side-bending using thenar eminence

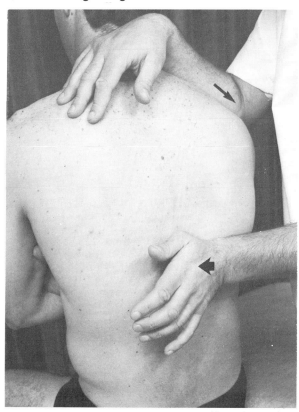

This hold performs the same function as the previous one but is a bit stronger as the operator is using the thenar eminence as the fulcrum to intoduce side-bending.

Side-bending articulation

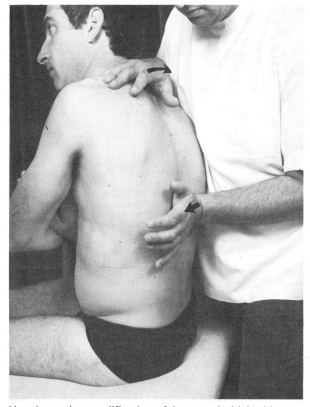

Here is another modification of the same hold. In this case the operator is pushing on the muscle bulk over the angles of the ribs rather than the spinous processes which are sometimes tender.

Hold back articulation

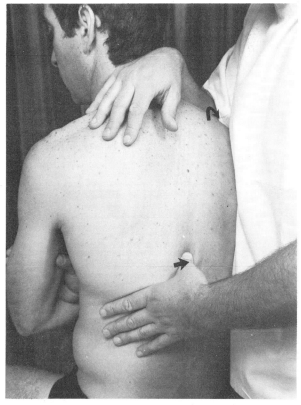

Although the basic hold is similar in this approach, the technique differs because the operator is holding back on the spinous process instead of pushing. This has the advantage that the spine below the fulcrum is largely prevented from movement and areas of irritability below the fixation point are unlikely to be upset.

Multiple direction articulation

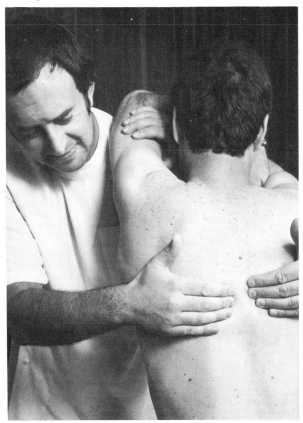

This hold allows the operator to introduce extension, side-bending, and rotation with only small changes of hand hold and alterations of body position. The patient must of course have healthy shoulder joints to make this technique feasible. The head is kept over the pelvis to aid stability and the spine is moved between the static position of the head and pelvis.

Extension and rotation articulation

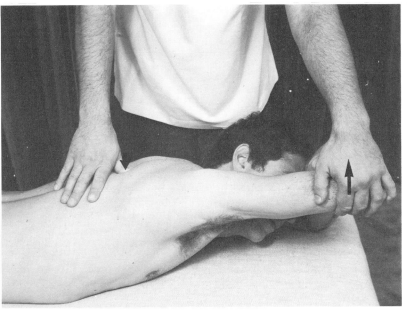

Extension and rotation can be induced in this position while the hand is holding back on the spinous process or on the transverse process or the angle of the ribs.

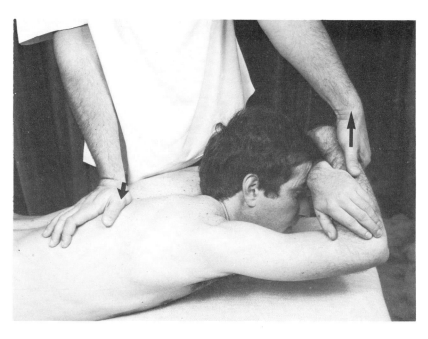

Extension articulation

Very strong extension is possible with this hold which can be modified to a gentle form of thrust if necessary, providing the amplitude is kept very low.

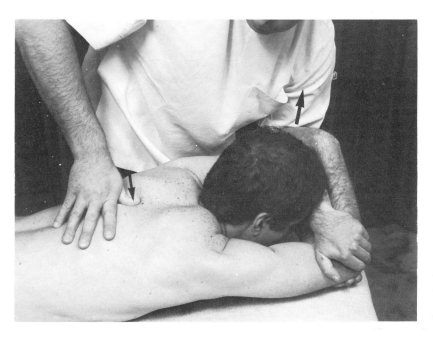

Specific articulation

This hold allows very specific articulation to individual segments although it is harder work on the operator than the previous holds.

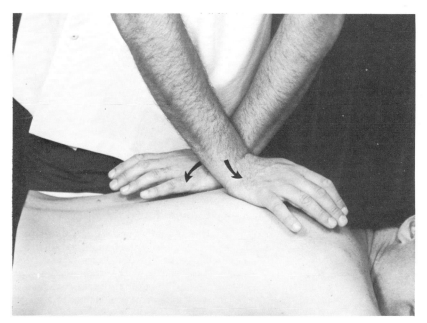

Prone dorsal thrust (1)

This thrust technique can be performed in several different ways. This particular approach uses the principle of side-bending to one side and rotation to the same side. This principle requires a higher amplitude than the other method using side-bending to one side and rotation to the other. The operator's left hand is inducing rotation by pressure towards the table while his right hand is inducing side-bending by pressure towards the patient's head.

79

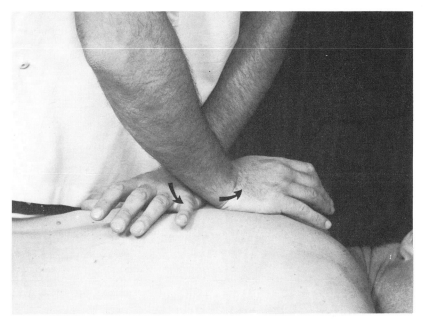

Prone dorsal thrust (2)

The leverage is fully taken up here. A careful study of this and the previous photo shows many subtle differences in wrist extension, variations of supination and pronation of the forearms etc.

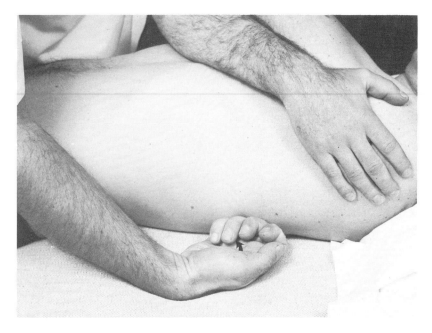

Supine dorsal thrust (1)

The operator's right hand is to be used as applicator in this picture. It is going to be placed under the patient who is lying supine. The thenar eminence and the bent fingers are placed either side of the spinous processes.

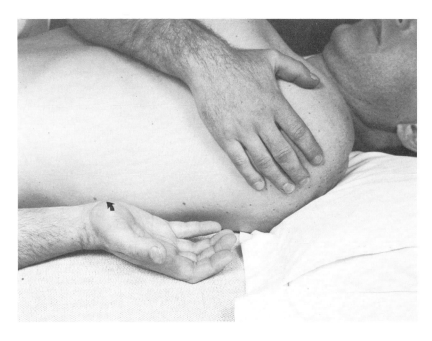

Supine dorsal thrust (2)

This alternative hand position is sometimes useful if the patient is particularly heavy or the operator's hand is uncomfortable in the previously shown method. Note that the wrist is held in slight extension to give the hand greater depth.

Supine dorsal thrust (3)

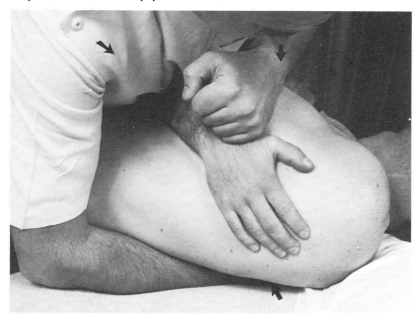

The underneath hand has been applied to the lamina of the chosen vertebra, the patient's crossed arms are gently compressed towards the table and then the thrust is applied with the operator's chest towards the patient's shoulders in the long axis of the humerus. At the same instant the applicator hand is pulled towards the pelvis and the wrist extended slightly more than at the start.

Supine dorsal thrust (4)

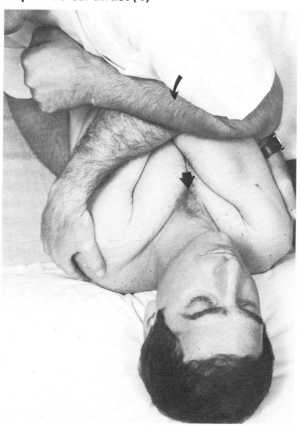

This picture may help to show more clearly the hold and direction of force.

Supine dorsal thrust (alternative hold)

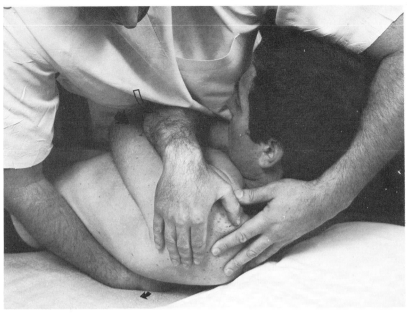

In a very flexible subject or where a flexion element is considered necessary, this alternative hold may be more useful.

Supine dorsal thrust (alternative hold)

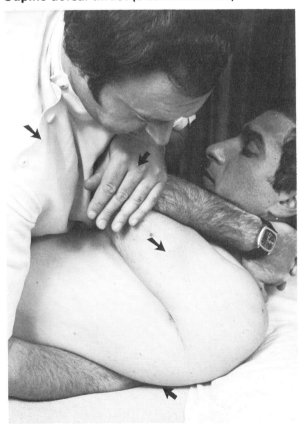

This alternative hold can be of use where the operator is working higher in the thoracic spine than with the previous method. The patient must have healthy shoulders and be able to get the hands into the clasped position behind the neck. A pad is sometimes necessary between the operator's chest and the patient's elbows.

Supine dorsal thrust

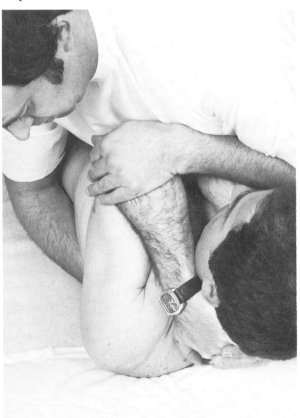

This alternative view may make the hold clearer to understand.

Supine dorsal thrust (alternative hold)

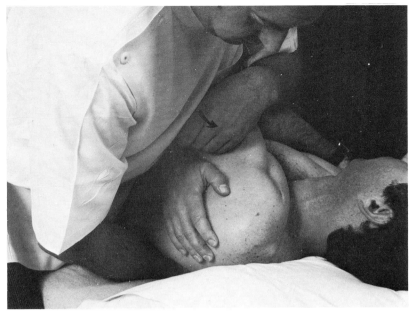

If the patient is very large or the operator is very small, then this approach where the applicator hand is put under from the nearside can be used.

Supine dorsal thrust (alternative hold)

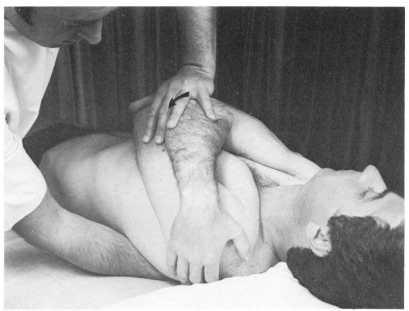

For very small patients and children this modification can be useful as the direction of force can be simply controlled by variations in hand pressure. Note that in all these modifications of the basic technique the basic combination of side-bending to one side and rotation to the other is used in combination with either flexion or extension. The use of these directions is not always obvious from the pictures as compression force is minimising the amount of leverage necessary and localising the forces.

83

Sitting dorsal thrust over fulcrum

Sitting dorsal thrust using traction

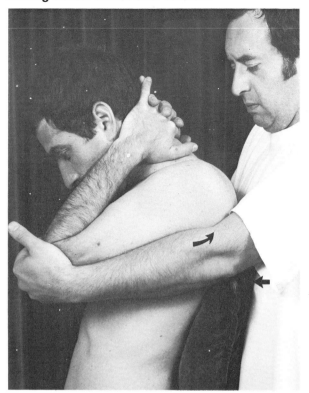

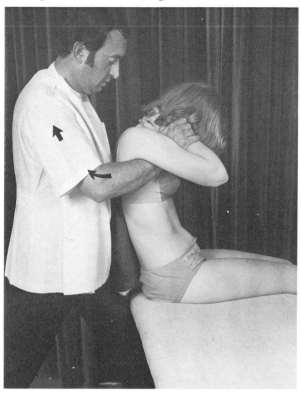

In this technique the operator is using a pad over his lower chest to localise the force to a particular area of the thoracic column above the pad. The patient's interlaced hands form a lever through which the force is applied, first into compression and then into a traction and flexion direction. This is combined with small amounts of side-bending and rotation to the opposite side as in the previous techniques.

This variation of the previous technique relies on the operator threading his hands through the patient's axillae, maintaining flexion in the thoracic curve and then applying the force in a direction of traction. A common fault in this modification is to allow the patient's shoulders to abduct too far and thus strain them. This is avoided if the operator keeps his forearms close to his sides.

Sitting dorsal thrust (alternative hold)

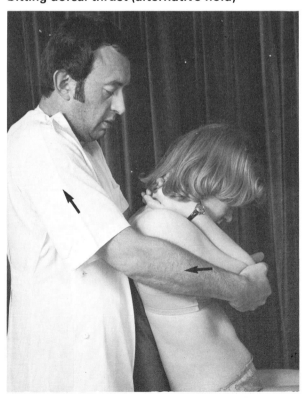

Here is another hold which is sometimes easier on patients, particularly if they have very mobile shoulders, as the adduction tends to limit the excessive movement and distracts the scapulae making the spinous processes more available for the thrust.

Sitting dorsal thrust (for rib)

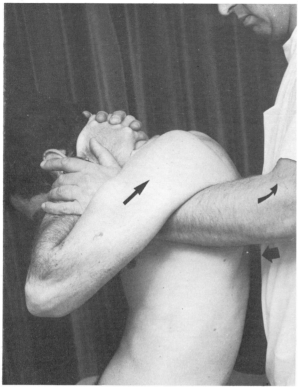

This shows a subtle variation in that the patient's body is rotated to his right and the fulcrum of the pillow is applied to the transverse process of the segment to be manipulated rather than the spinous process. This will of course tend to localise the force to the costo-transverse joint rather than the intervertebral joints. It can thus be used with breathing as a technique for specifically mobilising ribs as well as vertebral segments.

Sitting dorsal thrust (for rib)

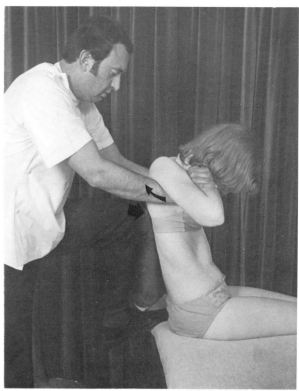

In this modification the operator's knee is being used as the fulcrum. This has the advantage of producing a semi-rigid fulcrum, but the inherent disadvantages of having to reach a long way for the hold and standing on one leg and thus being unstable have to be considered. If the segment to be manipulated is lower down, the operator can place his foot to the side and thus effectively "shorten" his leg, or the technique can be performed on a stool with cross-braces on which the foot can be placed.

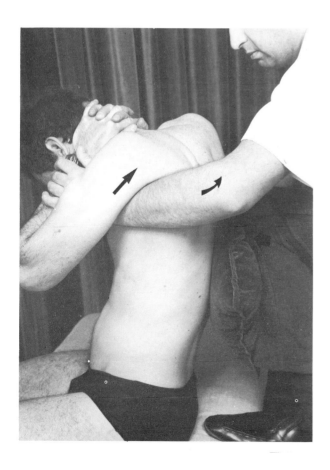

Sitting dorsal thrust (for rib)

Here the padded knee is shown applied to the transverse process or angle of a rib to localise the force to the costal element of a given level rather than the intervertebral element.

85

Sitting dorsal thrust from the front

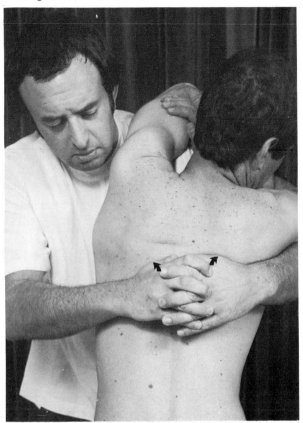

The operator has lifted the patient into a small degree of traction, applied side-bending to the patient's right, and by pulling towards himself with his left hand has rotated the patient's spine to the left. A small extension force with the thumbs will then suffice to gap the intervertebral joint at that level.

Prone dorsal thrust using head lever

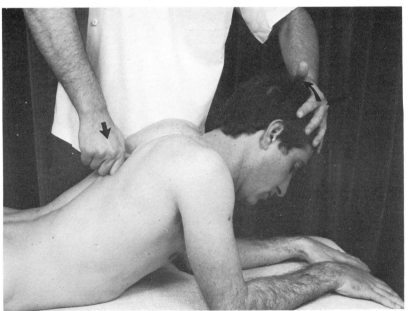

In this technique the patient's head is pushed gently into a compression direction towards the pelvis. The hand controlling the head can then apply side-bending to one side and rotation to the other which will be greatly amplified by the compression force. The operator's other hand is applied with the flexed first finger and thumb straddling the spinous process and applying a compression and rotation and side-bending force. The convergence of these forces will produce a gapping at the segment concerned if a small extra force is applied with the vertebral hand going into a small degree of supination or pronation.

Section C
Techniques for the shoulder and clavicle

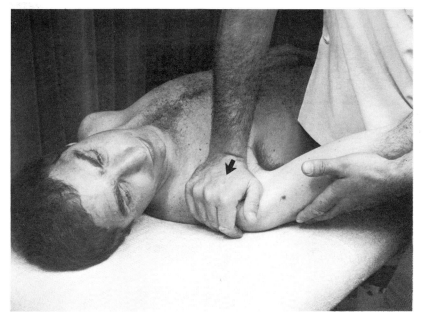

General hold for shoulder

This hold for general articulatory movements and specific soft tissue kneading techniques for the shoulder is particularly useful. It can be modified in many ways by the operator altering his position to introduce more abduction or less as the case requires. As the cross-fibre kneading is being performed the humerus can be rotated in the glenoid fossa to encourage the rotation movements, and flexion can be incorporated if desired as well. As the tissues in the front of the joint are accessible, and by reaching behind the joint the lateral and posterior muscles can be worked on also.

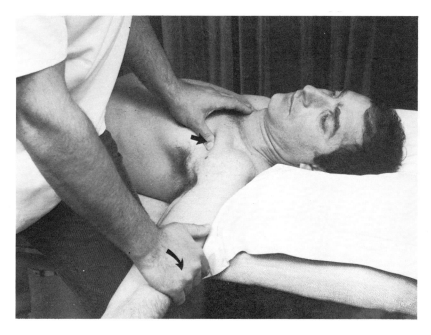

Stretch to pectoral muscles

This modified hold allows a particularly strong stretch to be applied to the pectoral muscles and their musculo-tendinous junctions. The arm can be rolled into external rotation as the technique is being performed and varying degrees of abduction are available.

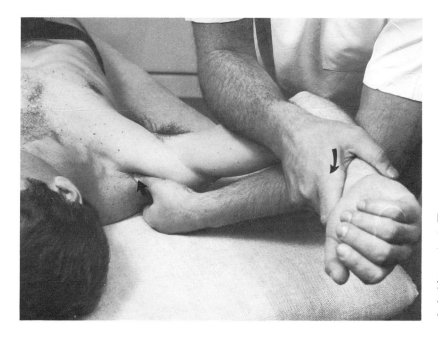

External rotation articulation

This hold demonstrates a specific articulatory procedure for the gleno-humeral joint as the acromio-clavicular joint is being fixed by the operator's left thumb. Repeated gentle stretching in varied degrees of flexion and abduction will reveal the optimum direction.

89

Close coupled hold for articulation

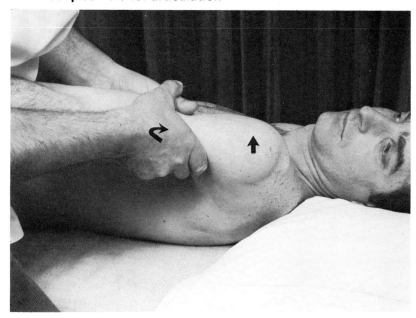

This hold allows the operator to exercise great control over the amplitude of movement at the shoulder joint and is not prone to produce undue stress. It allows the operator to use different degrees of traction and distraction at the same time as accessory movements of antero-posterior gliding.

Shoulder springing

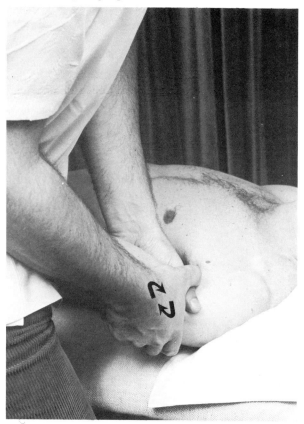

This hold, where the operator is holding right up in the axilla, gives very good control of all ranges of movement.

Side-lying external rotation

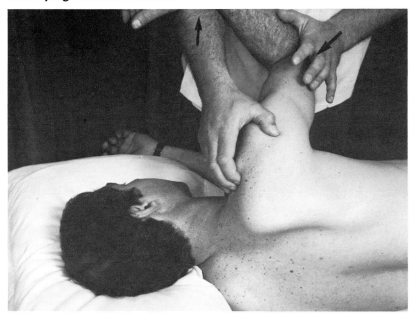

In this hold the operator is producing external rotation at the shoulder with varying degrees of flexion and abduction according to the position of his right forearm. His right hand is fixing on the clavicle and only gentle pressure is necessary on the patient's elbow to reach the limit of movement at the shoulder.

Side-lying internal rotation

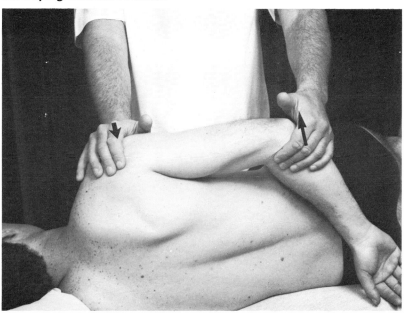

In this hold internal rotation is being emphasised. The operator's left hand is applying the force whilst the right hand is monitoring the effect at the shoulder joint. Stronger leverage can be applied by abducting the shoulder slightly before applying the rotation force.

Sitting articulation (all ranges)

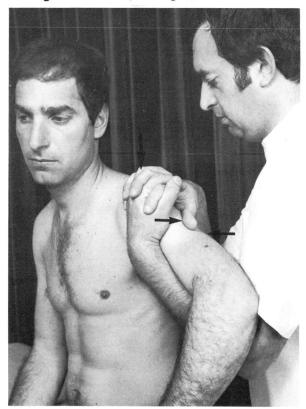

This complex hold allows flexion or extension in different degrees of abduction. Also traction can be applied by the operator holding back on the patient's scapula with his right forearm while he rotates his own body to the left. A distraction force can be brought into play by the operator pressing the head of the humerus towards the patient's pelvis. Varying degrees of rotation can be used also according to the initial placement of the patient.

Sitting articulation in traction (1)

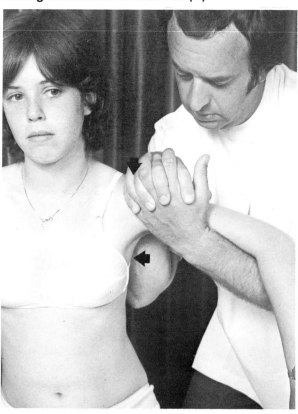

This anterior view of the technique shown in the previous picture shows the operator beginning to push on the scapula.

Sitting articulation in traction (2)

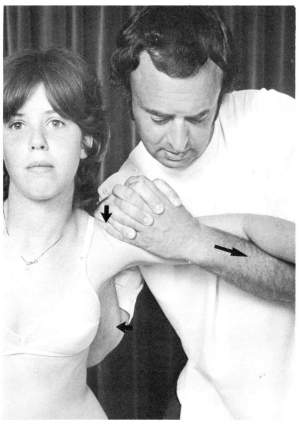

This shows the full hold applied. Note that the operator has rotated his own body to increase the effect of the technique.

Side-lying scapulo-humeral articulation

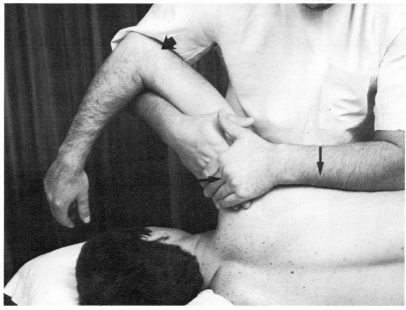

This hold is useful when treating the patient side-lying as the scapula is accessible to the operator for fixation and the humerus can be abducted in different ranges of rotation. The short leverages used here are much safer than long levers, particularly in elderly patients, or where there may be decalcification due to long-standing capsular adhesions and disuse atrophy.

Supine scapulo-humeral articulation

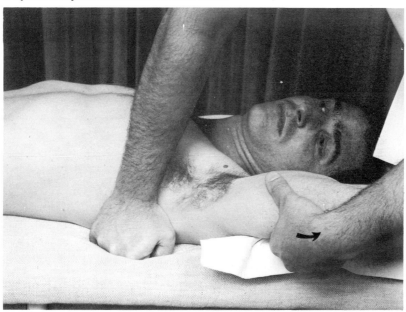

This hold is a very powerful stretch of the inferior part of the capsule of the shoulder and should be used with discretion. The operator's right hand is fixing the scapula and the other is applying traction, abduction and rotation internally or externally.

93

Side-lying traction

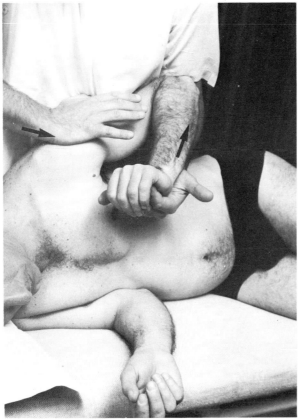

Side-lying traction in external rotation

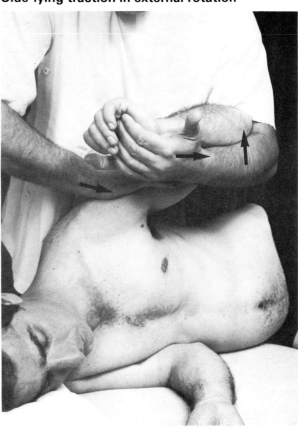

The use of traction can be amplified in this hold providing the patient's elbow is sound. The operator is clasping the patient's forearm between his flexed fingers and his elbow. The other hand is pushing the shoulder into a direction of traction and by the operator flexing and extending his left elbow, rotation can be achieved. If the operator flexes or extends his left shoulder this will produce flexion or extension of the patient's shoulder also. Greater degrees of abduction can be brought into play by the operator lifting his left shoulder. This hold allows nearly all the ranges of movement that might be desired to be produced.

Traction, abduction, external rotation, and flexion are shown here using the same hold as in the last technique.

Side-lying traction

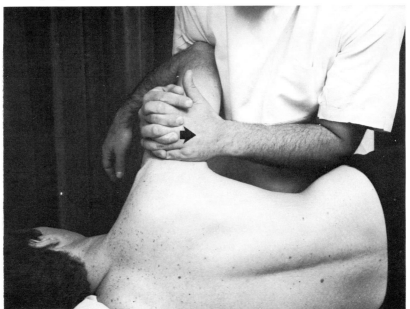

When standing in front of the patient this hold can be useful for producing traction with varying degrees of abduction and rotation internally or externally. Note that the patient's elbow is fixed against the operator's chest to form a pivot.

Side-lying scapulo-humeral traction

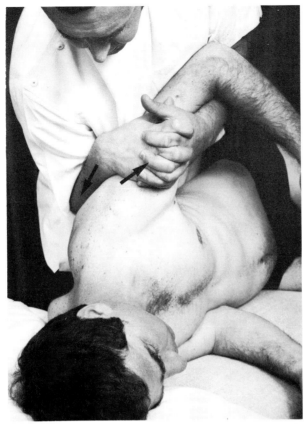

This hold allows the operator to hold back on the scapula at the same time as producing traction at the shoulder joint itself. Once again, different degrees of abduction and rotation can be used although with a little more awkwardness in this particular hold.

Supine traction in external rotation

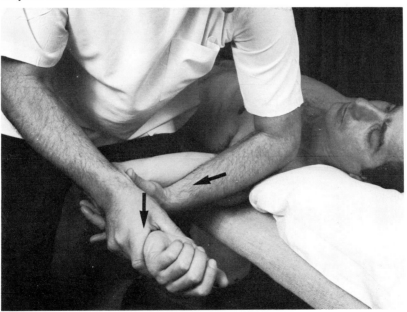

Using the patient's forearm as a lever, this hold allows traction and external rotation merely by the operator maintaining a steady hold on the patient's wrist, and pressure away from the patient's body in the bend of the elbow. This is of course a long lever technique and the usual caution should be observed.

Prone traction in external rotation

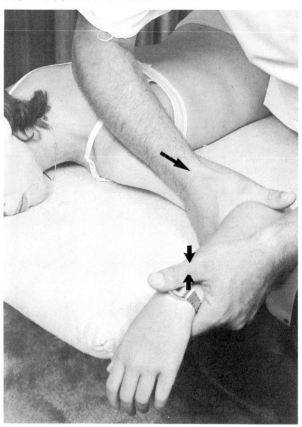

A prone position for traction and external rotation of the shoulder is shown here. Note that the operator is using his right forearm to stabilise the patient's scapula.

Supine traction in internal rotation

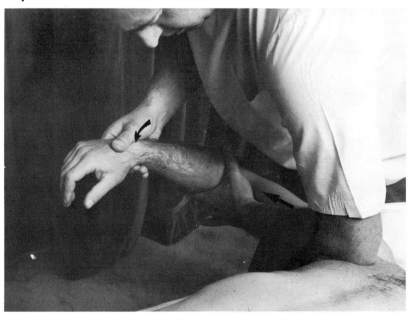

This hold shows the converse of the previous one, in that traction and internal rotation are being produced. Once again, different degrees of abduction are possible and various ranges of flexion or extension can be utilised.

Prone traction in internal rotation

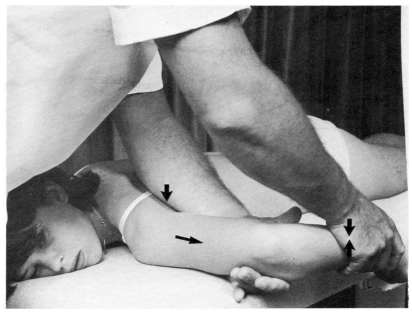

A supine position for applying traction and internal rotation is shown. Once again the operator is using his elbow to stabilise the scapula.

Sitting shoulder thrust technique

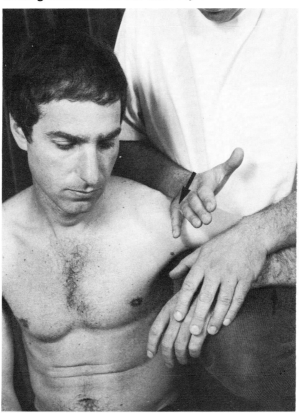

This technique is one of the few thrust techniques used on the shoulder joint itself. The arm is abducted to a comfortable degree and the patient encouraged to relax the shoulder as much as possible. A neutral position between internal and external rotation is found, and the operator then works his thrusting hand between the head of the humerus and the glenoid fossa. After a few preliminary trials a very short amplitude thrust is delivered in the direction of the patient's axilla. There is often an audible release and certainly a palpable change in the tissues. At the moment of the thrust a small increase in abduction can be used by the operator lifting his supporting leg slightly.

Antero-posterior gliding

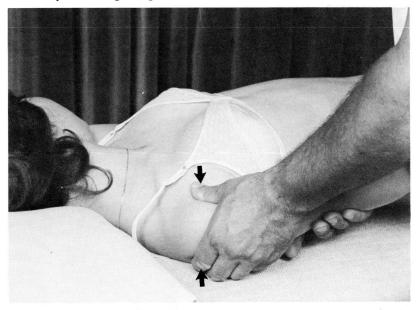

This hold is useful for the induction of antero-posterior movement in the shoulder joint. Care must be taken not to apply too much pressure over the long head of the biceps with the thumb.

Traction over a fulcrum

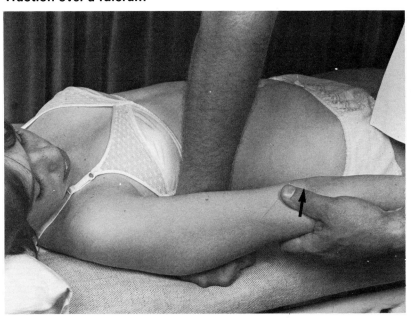

In this hold the operator has placed his right hand high in the axilla to form a fulcrum, and is pressing the patient's humerus towards the chest. This performs a strong traction movement on the gleno-humeral joint.

Traction and circumduction

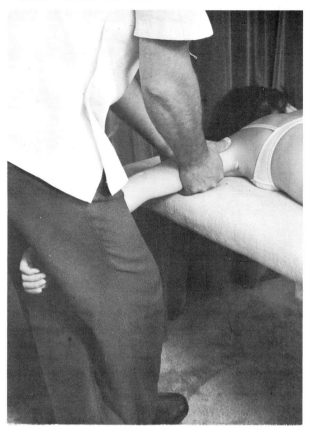

This hold can be used to allow the operator to have both hands free to work on the shoulder, and yet utilise a traction force. Note that the operator's feet are crossed. This means that as he leans back, he will clasp the wrist more firmly as the knees are straightened.

Traction and external rotation

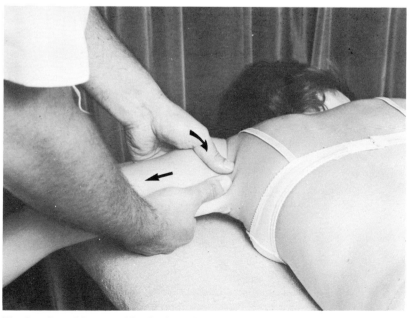

The hand position used in the last picture is shown here. External rotation is being used as well as traction via the wrist hold.

Clavicular articulation

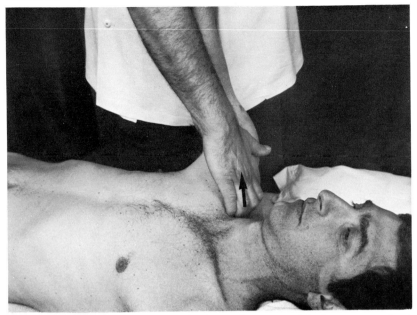

The clavicle features many times in the early osteopathic literature and yet relatively few techniques have been passed down for treatment to it and its articulations. This technique is for 'lifting' the clavicle. The operator's left hand (out of camera) is holding the patient's wrist and pulling it towards the ceiling. The right hand is clasping carefully behind the clavicle and lifting it forwards to stretch the clavipectoral fascia, the platysma and the sterno-clavicular joint. If the clavicle is firmly held in this position, the operator can then flex and elevate the patient's arm, thereby freeing the attachments of the clavicle.

Acromio-clavicular joint thrust (1)

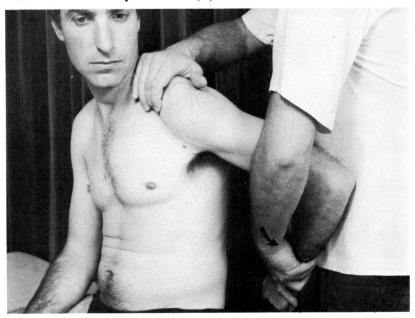

This picture and the next form a sequence for a thrust technique aimed at the acromio-clavicular joint. The patient's arm is internally rotated and extended and the clavicle is held in this position by the operator's right hand.

Acromio-clavicular joint thrust (2)

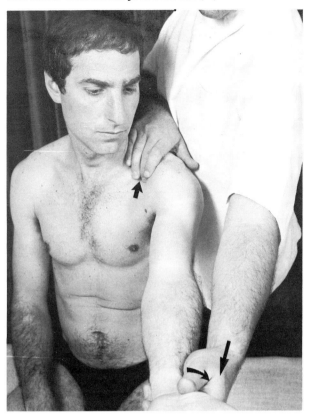

The position of the operator and the patient at the end of the thrust is shown here. The clavicle has been held back and the arm taken rapidly from extension and internal rotation, to flexion and external rotation. This sequence need not be performed violently, several repeated movements will usually achieve the same effect.

Acromio-clavicular joint thrust (3)

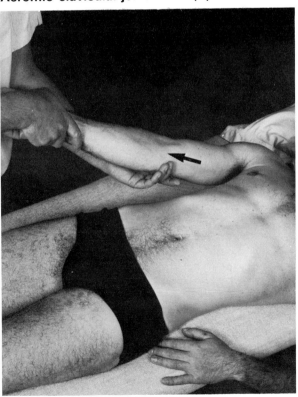

The acromio-clavicular joint can be reached in this hold by applying a short sharp tug to the arm whilst it is held in slight flexion and external rotation. It is important to ask the patient to side-bend his head to the affected side and rotate it the same way as well. This will help prevent undue traction trauma on the brachial plexus. Often several gentle trial pulls are necessary to find the optimum angle of pull.

Sterno-clavicular joint thrust

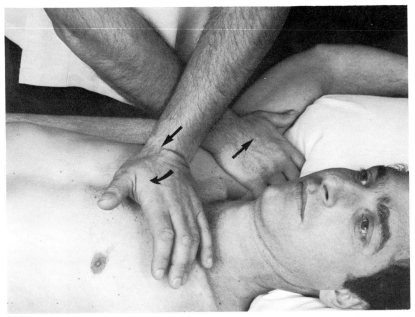

This complex technique is designed to adjust to medial and superior subluxations of the sterno-clavicular joint. The operator, having abducted and externally rotated the patient's arm is performing a combination of activities with both hands. The right hand is thrusting the distal third of the clavicle in the direction of the humerus. The left hand is pushing down (towards the patient's feet) on the sternal end of the clavicle, while at the same time prising the manubrium sternum away from the clavicle to give the joint room to re-align itself. The technique is performed with both hands acting simultaneously to achieve the maximum effect.

Clavicular stretch

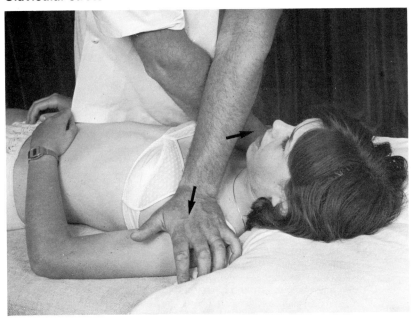

This hold can be used to stretch the sterno-clavicular joints bilaterally, and to apply a stretch to the acromio-clavicular joints as well.

Section D
Techniques for the elbow

Mobilisation in traction

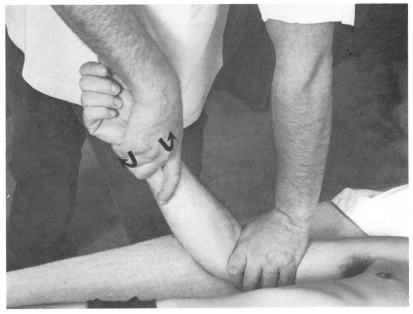

In this hold the elbow can be mobilised using traction. The operator's left hand is counter-fixing on the humerus while the other hand is pronating and supinating the radius and ulna under variable degrees of traction and flexion and extension. Note the hold above the patient's wrist to avoid placing undue stress on the wrist.

Lateral compartment stretch and thrust

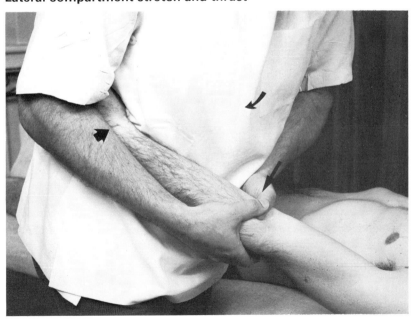

In this hold many different approaches become possible. The elbow can be mobilised in a medial and lateral gapping direction, as well as combining this with traction or compression if the operator leans back or forward respectively. The arrows show the usual direction of forces for thrusting the radio-humeral joint. Note that the operator's left arm is at right angles to the patient's arm, the operator has clasped the patient's hand into his side, and that whole body rotation is used to assist the thrust. The patient's forearm can be held in different degrees of pronation or supination as the needs of the case dictate. The direction of thrust in the approach to the radio-humeral joint is different from that to the humero-ulnar joint. The radio-humeral joint requires a thrust from medial to lateral and slightly anterior, i.e. towards the joint, whereas the humero-ulnar requires the thrust to be directly lateral or even slightly posterior.

Thrust to humero-ulnar joint

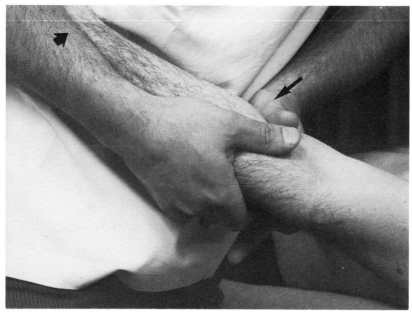

This view shows the direction of force necessary to produce gapping at the humero-ulnar joint. Note the angle of the operator's left forearm in relation to the patient's arm.

Thrust to radio-humeral joint

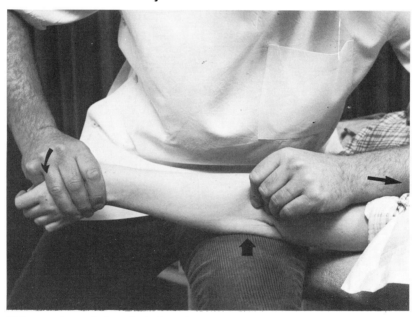

This complex technique is designed to gap the radio-humeral joint and employs several different contact points. The operator has placed the internally rotated arm of the patient across his thigh. The internal rotation must be maintained throughout the technique to ensure that the medial epicondyle is perpendicular to the lateral epicondyle and thus localise the force in the most effective way to the lateral side of the joint. The operator is fixing the patient's upper humerus with his left forearm to prevent anterior movement of the shoulder. He is palpating over the radio-humeral joint while the other hand produces pronation and supination to feel the optimum amount of tension in the joint with his left hand. The optimum is usually just short of full supination. The patient's elbow is maintained in a slight degree of flexion to allow some free play. The operator has his little finger in the palm of the patient's hand (this is optional) or the patient can be asked to clasp her own thumb in the palm of the hand to increase stretch on the extensor origin. The operator has applied ulnar deviation to the wrist to put the extensors on stretch. When all the forces have been localised by these combinations of levers the operator applies a small amplitude thrust to the patient's wrist towards the floor, while at the same time holding down the shoulder and plantar—flexing his foot to raise the fulcrum slightly. The tendency to allow the shoulder to fall into external rotation as the forearm is supinated should be avoided as this makes the technique ineffective.

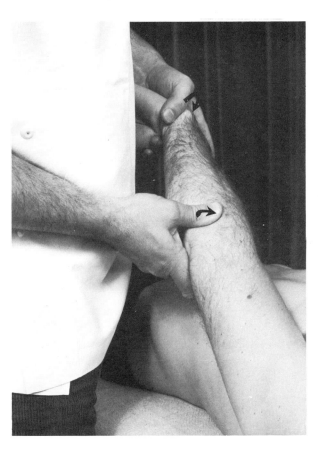

Modified 'mills' technique

This classical hold for manipulating the radio-humeral joint is often misused. The patient's forearm is pronated and the wrist held in almost complete flexion. The operator then takes the elbow from a few degrees of flexion into almost full extension at the same time as fully flexing the patient's wrist and thrusting with the thumb over the head of the radius. The operator places himself in such a position that the fully extended forearm meets his abdomen at the end of the thrust to avoid hyperextension. The obvious danger of hyperextension is however minimised even further if the operator introduces an element of lateral gapping into the elbow by pulling up (towards the ceiling) with his proximal hand. This serves to tighten the technique considerably and it is often found that the technique can be performed without even reaching full extension at all.

Radio-humeral gapping

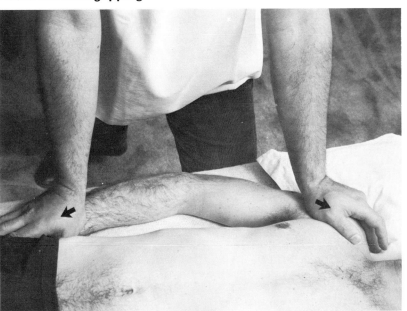

This hold is designed as a gapping technique for the radio-humeral joint. The patient's arm is placed in an easy, slightly flexed position resting on the table. The operator sets up an oscillating movement between his hands by rocking backwards and forwards. At the optimum point of tension the operator drives the humerus in a cephallic direction and the radius in a caudal direction. Although this method may not seem as effective as the previous techniques, it has the advantage that the elbow does not need to be in full extension which may not be possible for other reasons. Care must be taken that the hand thrusting on the humerus does not injure the long head of biceps which is vulnerable in this position. Quite considerable pre-loading of pressure is often necessary to make this technique effective.

Hold for humero-ulnar gapping (1)

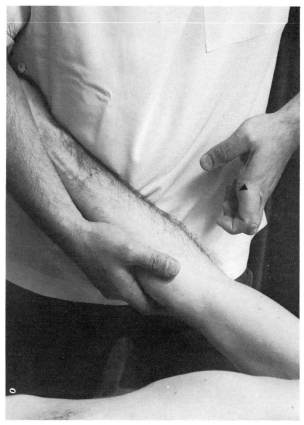

This shows the basic hold for a technique designed to mobilise the humero-ulnar joint where there is a diagnosis of a decreased carrying angle due to a joint dysfunction where the ulna tends to be held in adduction. Note the contact point which is the metacarpo-phalangeal joint which is applied to the lateral aspect of the proximal end of the ulna.

Hold for humero-ulnar gapping (2)

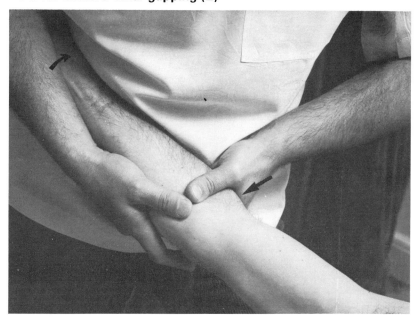

This picture shows the final position for the thrust to the ulna to increase the carrying angle. Note the use of operator body rotation to enhance the thrust and that the operator has placed the patient's forearm on the opposite side of his body than if he were to perform a thrust to decrease the carrying angle. The operator's thrusting arm is also nearly horizontal to direct the thrust towards the joint in question.

Medial gapping

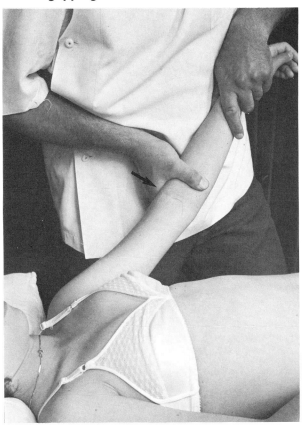

An alternative hold for applying a force to the lateral side of the elbow is illustrated here. This is not so strong or so controlled as the previous one.

General elbow articulation

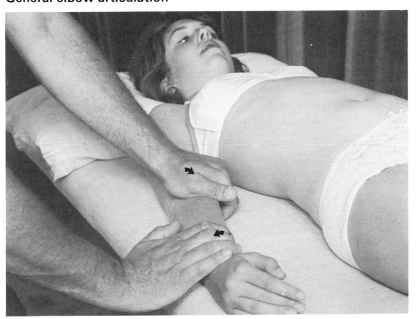

This "bone rolling" hold is useful for general mobilising of the elbow area. In this case the operator is supinating the forearm while holding back on the humerus.

Radio-humeral articulation

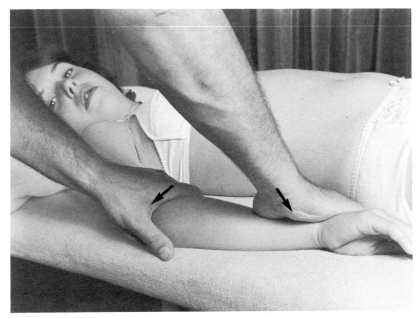

In this case the operator is holding back on the humerus and pronating the forearm. Sufficient tension can be produced in this hold to specifically direct the force to the radio-humeral joint with or without traction if necessary.

Section E
Techniques for the wrist

General wrist articulation (1)

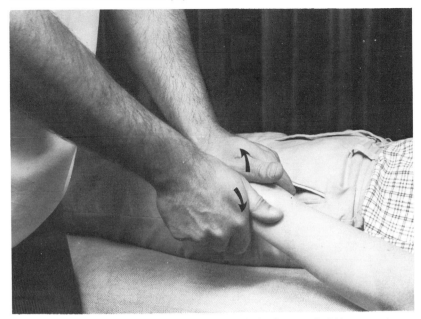

The wrist can be mobilised using this hold with the forearm held in pronation or supination. The operator is alternately ulnar and radially deviating his own wrists to produce a shearing force at the wrist. This can be directed to any area of the wrist by slightly altering the angle of approach.

General wrist articulation (2)

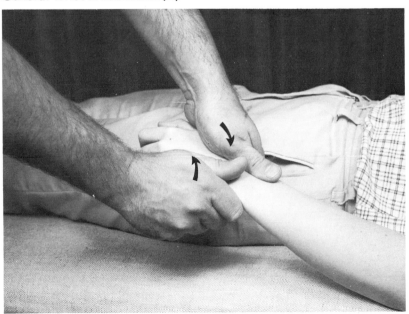

This shows the other extreme of movement of the previous hold. The picture shows the operator's hands remote from his body for clarity, whereas the technique would be best performed with them closer to him to increase the power available if necessary.

Carpal tunnel stretching (1)

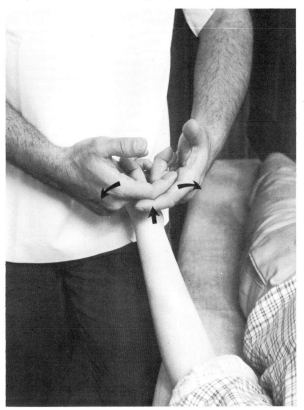

The hand position to stretch the carpal tunnel is shown here. The operator's crossed fingers are applied to the dorsum of the wrist and the thumbs to the palmar aspect.

Carpal tunnel stretching (2)

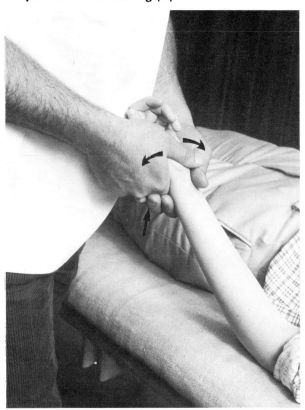

The hands here are applied so that the carpal tunnel can be stretched. Note that the stretch can be enhanced if the operator simultaneously ulnar and radially deviates his hands so that the stretch is in a diagonal direction.

Carpal tunnel stretching (3)

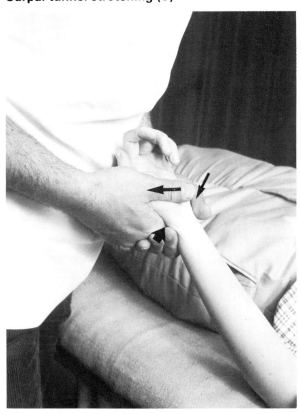

An extreme of stretch is shown here. Note that the operator has leaned forward to increase the effect of the hand position.

Traction and articulation

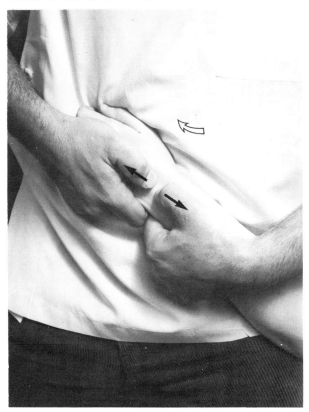

In this hold the operator has turned his back on the patient and by pivoting from his left to right, rotating his body away from the patient, he has placed the wrist on traction. The thumbs can then be used to localise the force to a specific joint or area whilst under traction and antero-posterior movement can be introduced as well.

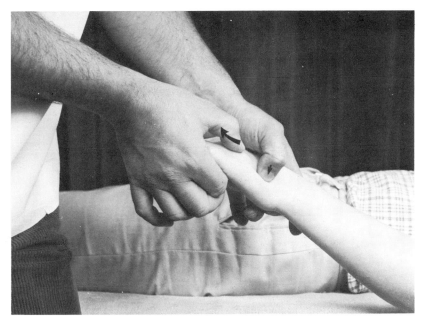

Metacarpo-phalangeal articulation (1)

This hold can be used to produce specific movement to the metacarpo-phalangeal joints. Here dorsiflexion is being induced under traction if desired.

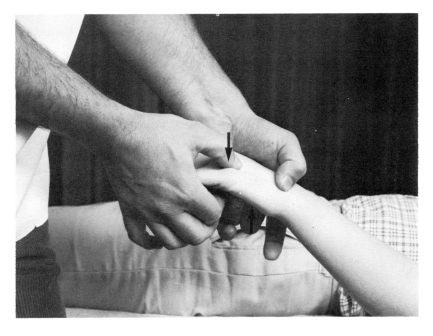

Metacarpo-phalangeal articulation (2)

This shows the converse movement to the previous picture in that traction and palmar flexion are being introduced. Rotation, abduction and adduction or any combination of movements can be made with this hold also.

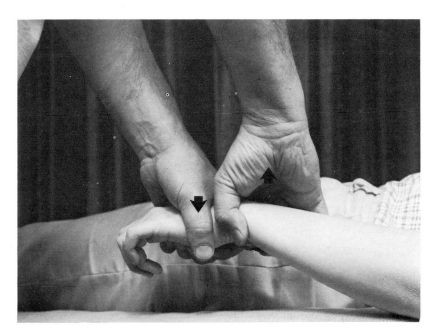

Shearing carpal rows (1)

Shearing movements of the proximal row of the carpus on the radius and ulna, or the distal row on the proximal row can be used in this hold.

Shearing carpal rows (2)

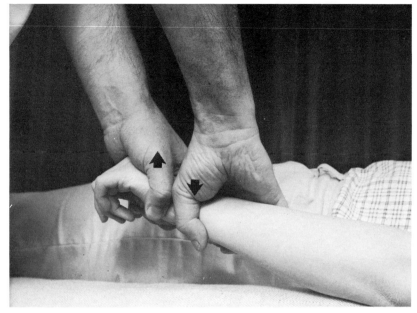

This shows the converse movement to the previous picture.

Specific thrusting to carpals in pronation

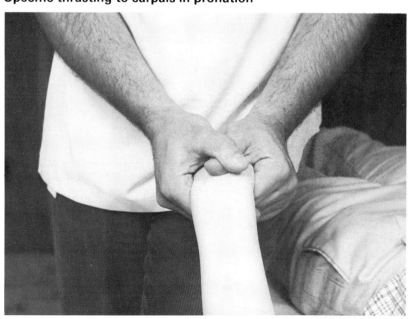

The starting position for specific thrusting techniques to individual wrist bones is shown here. From this position different degrees of abduction, adduction, flexion, extension and composite movements can be introduced prior to performing a thrust in a predetermined direction.

Specific thrusting to carpals in supination

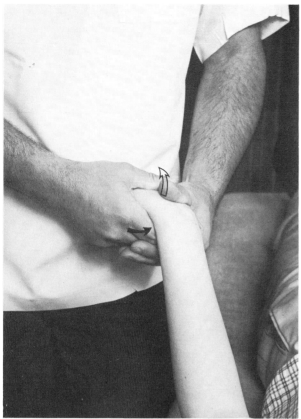

This shows the general position for thrusting individual wrist bones from the dorsal to the palmar aspect. Variations in direction of thrust must be introduced according to the specific carpal bone being worked. Specific directions for each individual bone are not shown as the subtle variations that the individual anatomy dictates makes pictorial representation very difficult.

Thrust to trapezium joint to first metacarpal

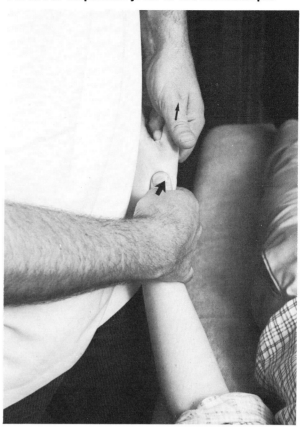

The one individual bone which is not too difficult to demonstrate pictorially is the trapezium in its articulation with the first metacarpal. The operator is holding firmly over the trapezium and whilst applying traction to the thumb, is gently rotating the first metacarpal back and forth and applying extension. When the optimum position is found a very small emphasis of the thumb pressure on the trapezium will effect a gapping.

Interphalangeal joint gapping

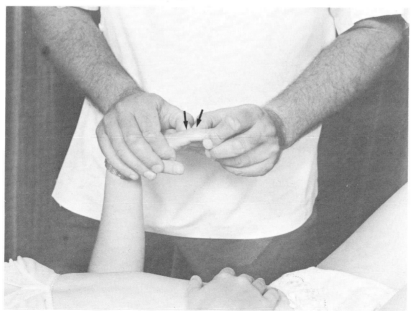

The inter-phalangeal joints can be manipulated with this hold. Note that the joint is held in slight flexion, and then a lateral force is applied to specifically stretch the lateral ligament, or a specific part of the capsule.

117

Section F
Techniques for the hip

Hip articulation in internal rotation and flexion

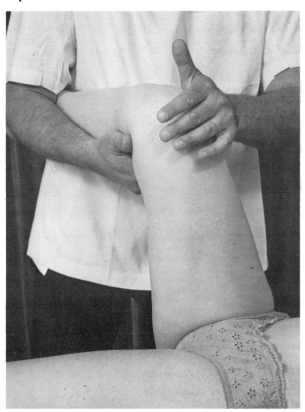

This general hold can be used for mobilising the hip joint in ranges of flexion, internal rotation, adduction and abduction. Some stress is put upon the knee which must be minimised if it is uncomfortable.

Hip articulation in external rotation

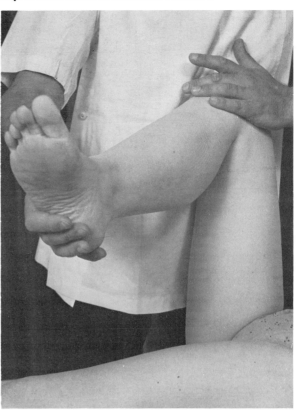

This hold is useful for introducing external rotation in different degrees of flexion and extension. The knee must be protected from undue stress in this technique also.

Hip internal rotation 'stress' technique

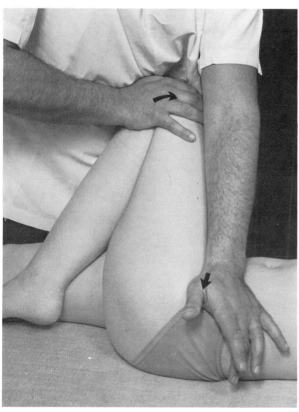

This hold can be used where there is a resistance to internal rotation which is deemed to emanate from soft-tissue restriction rather than arthrosis. The hip is taken to the limit of internal rotation and held there under a degree of sustained pressure until a sense of release is felt. This can take up to 20 or 30 seconds. As this release is felt, a small stressing of the position can be introduced. This is hardly a thrust, but nevertheless could be classified as a low velocity thrust technique.

Strong internal rotation in flexion

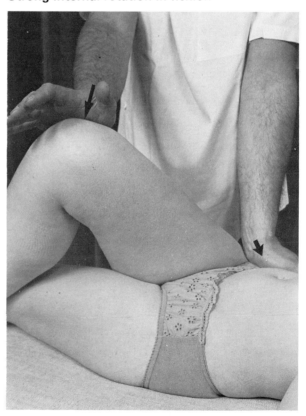

This shows how the operator can apply internal rotation in adduction from the same side as the affected hip. Note that in this picture the patient's ankle is placed lateral to the other leg to produce stronger adduction. The operator's hand applied to the patient's anterior superior iliac spine is sometimes uncomfortable and then a pad can be used.

121

External rotation 'stress' technique

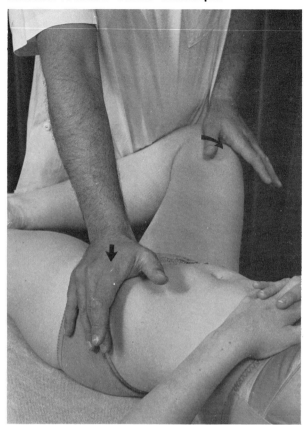

If the hip is limited and uncomfortable in external rotation, this hold can be used as a stress technique to increase the range. Once again this is not a thrust technique, the hip is held in a stressed position until a sense of give is acquired. This may well take up to 30 seconds, then the movement is stressed a little further as the muscles "give way". The patient's ankle need not be placed on the opposite knee, it could be placed medial to the other knee, or medial to the other tibia in less flexible cases.

Side-lying general articulation hold

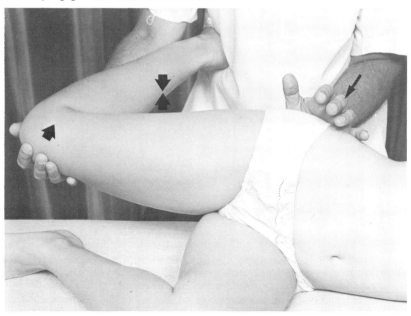

This hold allows very good control of the hip joint. Internal and external rotation can be induced as well if desired, as can adduction and abduction. Varying degrees of flexion of the knee will direct the force to the muscles, ligaments, capsule or joint itself.

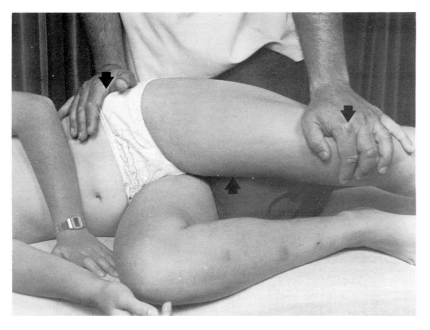

Traction over a fulcrum

This hold is used to induce a true traction in the hip joint. The operator is using his own knee as a fulcrum as high in the groin as possible. The knee is maintained in extension to apply a force across the joint via the fascia lata, the pelvic hand is used to hold back on the ilium and pressure is applied with both hands. This serves to lift the head of the femur out of the acetabulum.

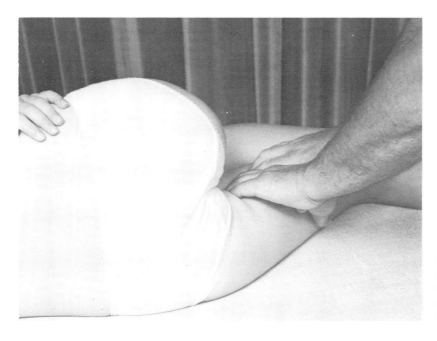

Cross-fibre kneading to adductors

This position is useful for applying cross-fibre kneading to the adductors in the thigh. It allows the operator to get right up to the pubis without too much difficulty.

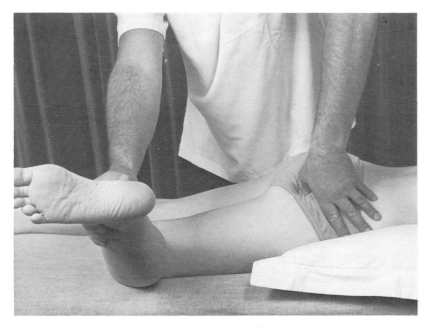

Pyriformis inhibition

Several authorities cite the Pyriformis muscle as being a common site for irritation of the sciatic nerve. This hold can be used for two ways of influencing the Pyriformis. With firm pressure over the muscle belly, the hip is stretched into internal rotation, thereby putting the muscle on stretch. In this case the operator's thumb is being used to apply inhibition at the same time. This same hold can be used to apply a muscle energy technique, where the operator asks the patient to actively externally rotate the hip against the resistance of the operator's hand, after several seconds the patient is asked to relax and the hip will have been found to be able to internally rotate further due to the reflex inhibition of the external rotators after contraction. This can be repeated several times until the desired result is achieved.

Pyriformis inhibition

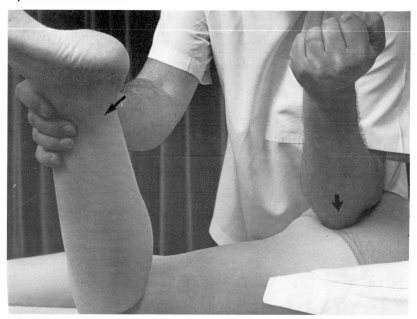

Here is shown an alternative method of applying inhibition to Pyriformis which is obviously much stronger. Note that the patient's pelvis is thrown into slight preliminary flexion by placing a pillow under the anterior superior iliac spines. This method is useful for the operators who find the use of the thumb impossible due to instability of their own joints.

Section G
Techniques for the sacro-iliac joints

Sacro-iliac articulation (1)

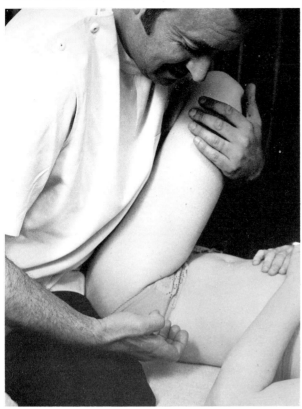

This shows one useful hold for testing the range and quality of movement in the sacro-iliac joint. A common configuration for the palpating hand is shown.

Sacro-iliac articulation (2)

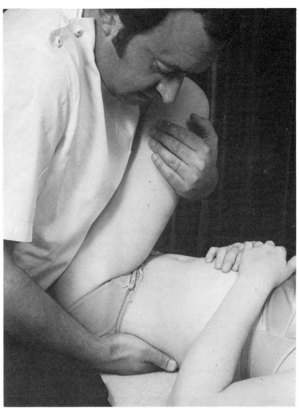

The hold is here applied to test or mobilise the sacro-iliac joint. Note that the operator is sitting on the edge of the table, although this is not always convenient. The patient's hip can be circumducted, or internally or externally rotated from this position, with greater or lesser degrees of adduction, flexion or abduction as the case dictates.

Sacro-iliac articulation (3)

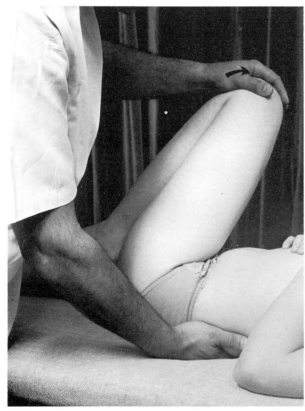

This alternative hold is a useful diagnostic approach. Although the range of free movement in the sacro-iliac joint is very small, the quality of free movement is very easy if the joint is placed in a neutral position. In this hold the operator can oscillate the hip into adduction and feel this free movement very easily.

Sacral springing (1)

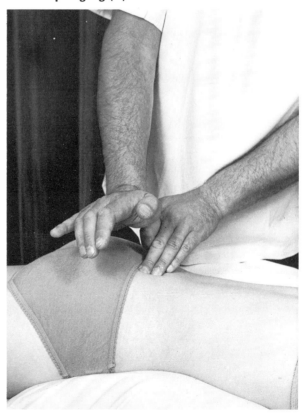

This shows a palpating hand applied to the sulcus of the sacro-iliac joint just medial to the posterior superior iliac spine. The other hand is about to be applied to the sacrum. In many cases the amount of free movement in the joint is so small that the mere weight of the hand is sufficient to obliterate the range. In this case it is better to apply and remove the hand rather than to press more and less firmly.

Sacral springing (2)

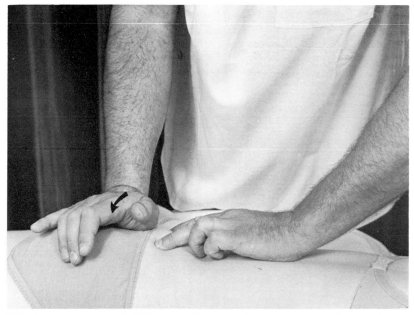

This shows a common hold for assessing sacro-iliac movement. The sacral hand is flexing and releasing the sacrum, while the palpating hand is assessing the range and quality of movement using the tips of the first two fingers. The rate of oscillation of the sacral pressure may have to vary from case to case, sometimes a very rapid gentle oscillation will give the best feedback.

Sacral springing (3)

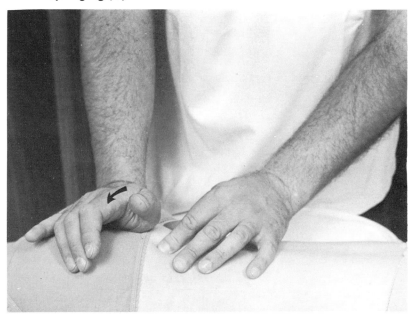

In this picture an alternative palpating hold is used where the operator is using the first finger and thumb to palpate as the sacrum is flexed and released. It is often easier to assess quality of movement on the release of pressure by feeling the recoil in the tissues.

Springing the ilium postero-anteriorly

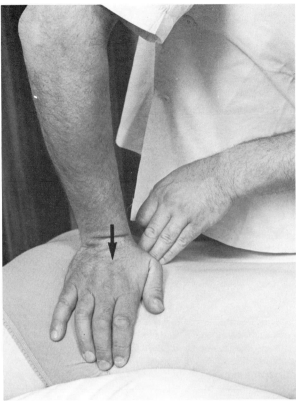

The operator's left hand is palpating the sacro-iliac sulcus while the right hand is pressing the ilium directly anteriorly. In most cases this will lead to very little actual range of movement in the sacro-iliac joint although it will give a useful differentiation between actual joint movement and soft-tissue spring around the joint. In other words the operator is approaching the joint from a "wrong" direction so that when the "right" direction is reached it should have a sense of "give" which is much more obvious.

Springing the ilium infero-superiorly

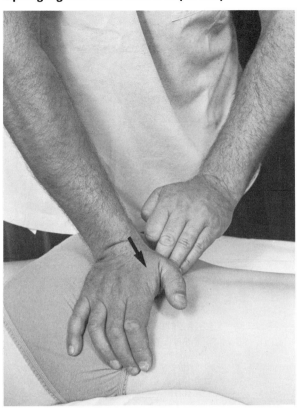

As in the last picture, the operator is approaching the joint in a "wrong" direction to assess the spring in the surrounding tissues before attempting to move the ilium on the sacrum in a sliding direction.

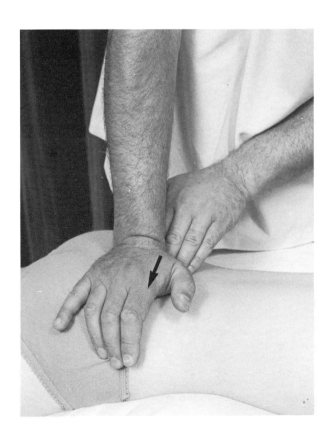

Springing the ilium along the joint

In this picture the operator is attempting to align the gliding force with the plane of the joint as determined by the previous pressures in the "wrong" directions which should make the "right" direction more easily felt.

129

Springing over the fifth lumbar

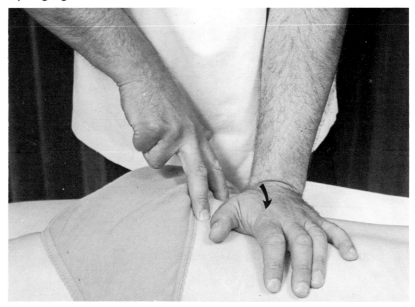

In many cases it is useful to assess the range and quality of movement of the lumbar spine on the sacrum, and the relationship of lumbar movement to the sacro-iliac joints. This hold will make this assessment easier. The operator is pressing gently from posterior to anterior on the spinous processes of the L5 and L4 segments whilst palpating the sacro-iliac movement. This will also of course show the reactivity of the lumbar spine to direct pressure which may be of help in determining the best approach to treatment of a case of instability due to ligamentous laxity, spondylolisis or spondylolisthesis.

Differential hip/sacro-iliac/lumbar test

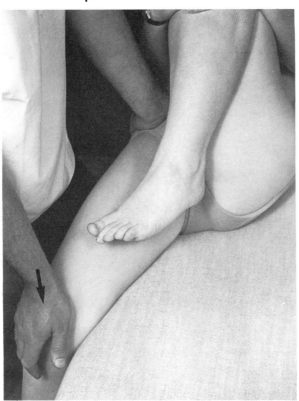

This hold serves a number of purposes. Its inclusion here is in its capacity to help in the differentiation of symptoms originating in the sacro-iliac joint as against the lumbar joints. The patient is holding her own knee, thereby flexing the lumbar spine, if symptoms are produced on extending the affected side, they may well be due to sacro-iliac dysfunction. However, if symptoms are obliterated when the patient holds the knee, they are probably due to a lumbar cause as extension of the affected side has little effect on the lumbar spine locked by the patient's own effort. This test will naturally show up excessive tightening in psoas and the hip flexor muscles as well as the operator will not be able to extend the hip as far as expected.

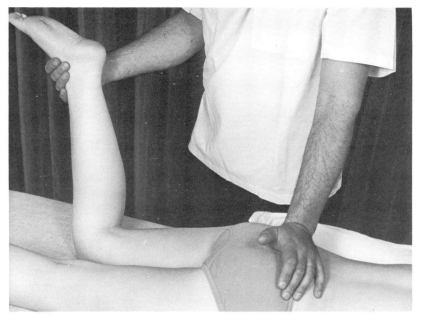

Sacro-iliac articulation (1)

This basic hold can be used once again for a number of different purposes. The operator can either hold on the sacrum or over the posterior superior, or posterior inferior iliac spine. The pressure with this hand can be directed in several different directions, and can be accompanied by a thrust if necessary. The leg hand can be used to circumduct the knee, thereby rotating the hip, and flexing the knee thereby putting the hip flexors on tension if desired.

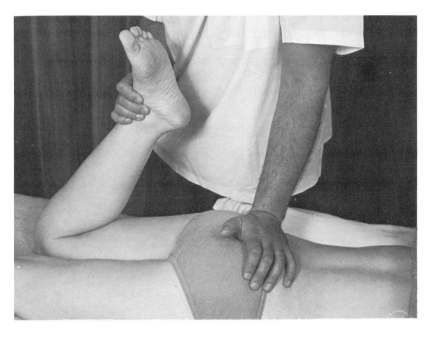

Sacro-iliac articulation (2)

In this picture the patient's knee is partially flexed to put the flexors on stretch. The operator is pressing directly towards the table with the sacral hand and by assessing the tension in the sacro-iliac joint from the resistance to movement he can specifically mobilise the joint by balancing the forces between the two hands.

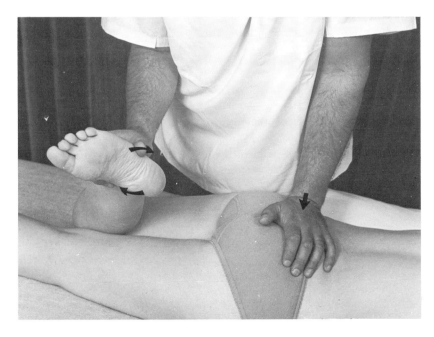

Sacro-iliac articulation (3)

Here the operator has externally rotated the patient's hip thereby tending to rotate the ilium in a backwards direction. This force is reinforced by the operator pressing the sacrum towards the table and in a gapping direction to mobilise the sacro-iliac joint. Firm articulation near the limit of range can act as a very efficient method of increasing mobility. Note that the patient's hips have been elevated on a pillow to attempt to obliterate some of the lumbar lordosis which is often uncomfortable if this precaution is not taken.

131

Sacro-iliac articulation (4)

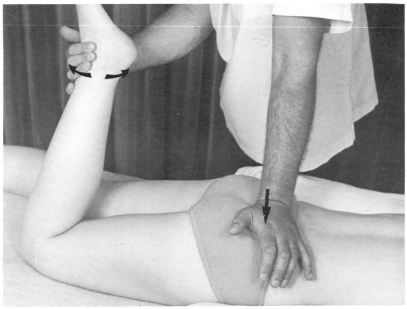

In this case the operator is standing on the opposite side to the affected joint. The hand pushing on the posterior superior iliac spine is directed towards the table from the mid line outwards, whilst the other hand is circumducting the knee until the sense of tension is felt at the sacro-iliac joint when a little further stress of the movement can be applied. The key to all the varieties of hold using this particular technique is the firmness of pressure on the sacrum or the ilium. They will not work to any great extent if this pressure is not firm. Note that any variation in the patient's position on the table will influence the technique. For example, if the patient's hands are above her head, Latissimus Dorsi is on more tension and there will be greater pull up on the pelvis. Rotation of the head towards the affected side will increase the tension on the joint whereas rotation away will diminish it due to variation in pull on Trapezius etc.

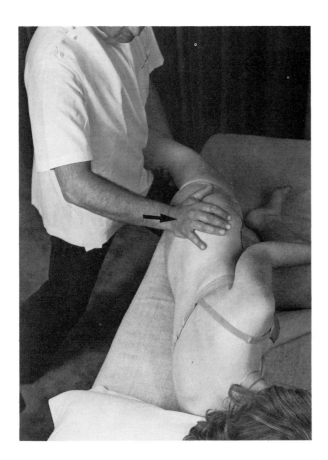

Sacro-iliac/lumbar test

This hold can be used for testing for differentiation between sacro-iliac pain and lumbar pain. The patient holds her own knee and hip in flexion thereby tending to put the lumbar spine into flexion and limit movement there. As the operator extends the other hip he tests for production of pain. If the pain is produced with the lumbar spine relatively fixed, the most likely source is the sacro-iliac. If however there is pain when the patient releases the leg and not when it is held, the source is most likely the lumbar spine. Of course if there is pain in both situations it is possible that either the lumbar spine or the sacro-iliac joint is at fault and the test is little help. The position can be used also for mobilising the sacro-iliac into a more forward rotation, if the diagnosis is of a "posterior" innominate.

Direct thrust to ilium forwards (1)

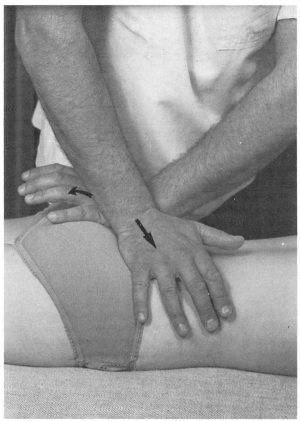

In this picture the operator has applied pressure over the posterior superior iliac spine with one hand, and over the sacrum with the other. The optimum angle for releasing the joint has been previously determined by springing. The operator then holds the sacrum firmly and applies a thrust along the line of the iliac crest to guide the innominate forwards.

Direct thrust to ilium forwards (2)

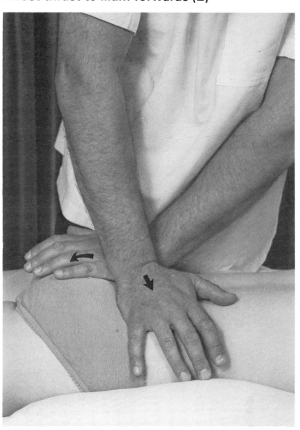

This shows the completed technique position of the previous hold. Note that the operator's thrusting hand has moved closer to the table and that the sacral holding hand has in fact slightly increased its movement towards the feet.

Direct thrust to ilium forwards (3)

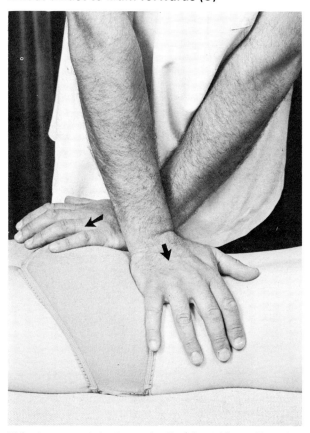

This shows a subtle change in direction of force. Note that the sacral hand has pulled the sacrum away from the ilium to induce a gapping force and assist the technique.

133

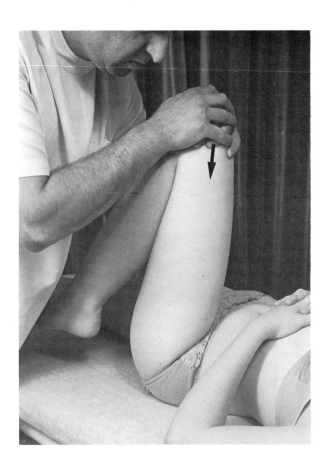

Thrust to gap sacro-iliac joint forwards

As the acetabulum is anterior and inferior to the axis of movement of the sacro-iliac joint, any pressure vertically towards the table will tend to push the ilium into a forward rotation direction. This would seem to be contrary to expectation but a study of the anatomy will prove the point. The hip needs to be held in slight internal rotation to tension the capsule and the "Y" ligament. The thrust must be fairly fast to break the fixation before the pelvis rotates from the pressure. If the hip is flexed beyond 90 degrees then the pull of the extensor muscles will negate the effect of the technique.

Thrust forwards using patient's muscle action

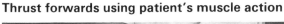

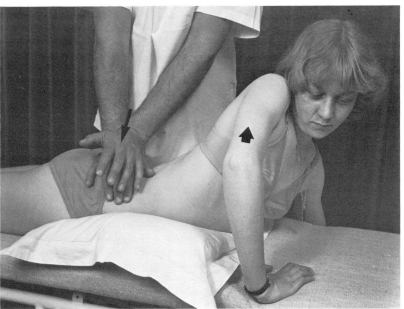

This technique utilises isometric contraction by the patient to attempt to rotate the spine off the table and at the same time the operator maintains pressure on the posterior superior iliac spine. When the optimum tension is sensed, the operator can make a small thrust. Variations in the amount of side-bending will alter the effectiveness of the technique. One important requirement is that the operator maintains sufficient pressure to keep the anterior of the pelvis in contact with the table to prevent excessive extension of the spine when performing the thrust.

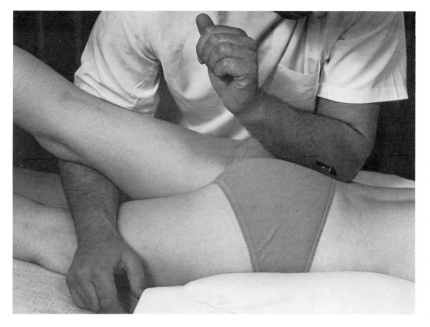

Long lever sacro-iliac thrust forwards using elbow

In this technique the operator is using the tension of the flexor apparatus of the hip, and the hip capsule to pull the innominate backwards. The hip is also adducted to put the fascia lata on tension. The thrusting part of the arm is, in this case the medial aspect of the operator's elbow. The point of the elbow is to be avoided as it is very uncomfortable for the patient and no more effective for the operator. The thrust is directed along the crest of the ilium.

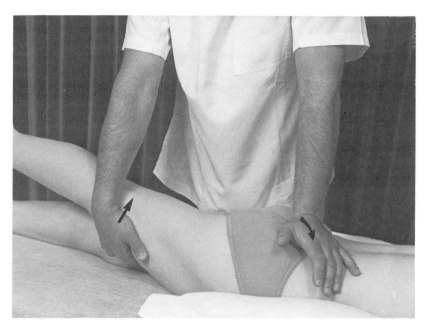

Long lever sacro-iliac thrust forwards using heel of hand

This technique employs the same principles as the previous one. The difference in the hold here means that the operator stands on the opposite side of the table to the affected side. The patient's thigh is lifted off the table until the tension is optimum at the posterior superior iliac spine, assisted by the operator adducting the thigh and internally rotating it. The thrust is then directed along the line of the crest to break any fixation in an "anterior" direction.

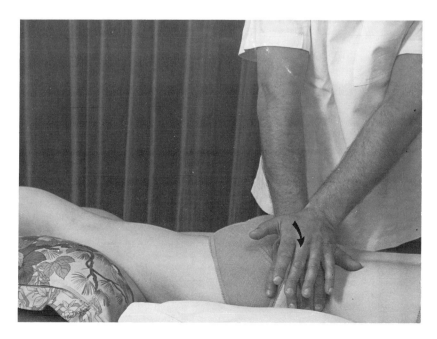

Sacro-iliac thrust forwards using pillow and both hands

If the operator is small, or the patient's leg is very heavy, it can be propped up on pillows, and the force therefore concentrated by the operator at the thrust point with both hands.

135

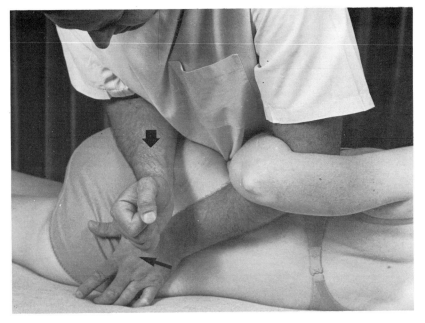

Side-lying sacro-iliac thrust forwards to lower joint

This technique for a "posterior" innominate uses the same basic position as the conventional lumbar side-lying thrust technique but with several major differences. The operator's right hand is rotating the patient's pelvis to the patient's right, and therefore tending to push the patient's right ilium backwards. However the operator is holding back on the right posterior superior iliac spine (the one nearest the table), and as the thrust is applied to the upper hip area, the lower hand thrusts the ilium downwards and forwards. This needs a fine appreciation of tension and forces to be successful, but with practice, can be a useful technique to avoid changing the patient's position excessively. It has the disadvantage that as a lot of leverage is being applied through the lumbar spine, it is difficult to be sure that the technique is being absolutely specific.

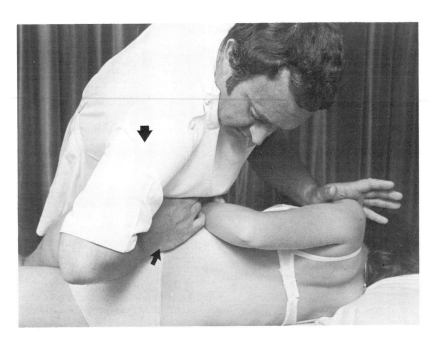

Side-lying sacro-iliac thrust forwards to upper joint

Using the basic lumbar side-lying position, and a degree of compression, this modification is very useful for thrusting directly forwards on the posterior superior iliac spine.

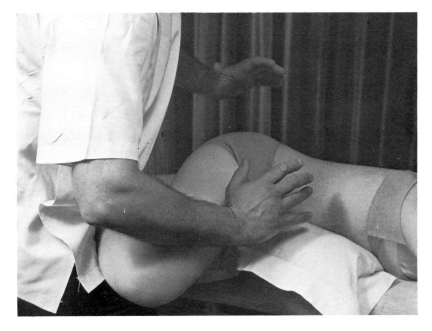

Prone sacro-iliac thrust backwards (1)

In the situation where the operator decides that the sacro-iliac joint needs to be mobilised into a "posterior" direction, as it is fixed in a relatively "anterior" direction, this technique can be used. The patient's hip is abducted and flexed and externally rotated. The tibia is resting across the operator's flexed thighs, and he is about to place his right hand under the anterior superior iliac spine. The left hand is about to be placed over the ischial tuberosity and the hip bone is therefore firmly sandwiched between the hands.

Prone sacro-iliac thrust backwards (2)

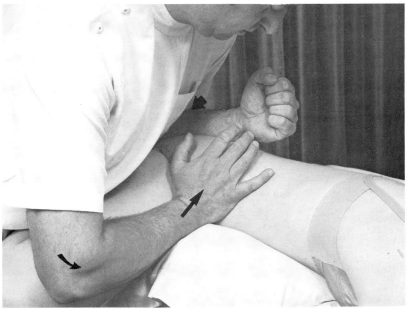

Here the hands are applied, and the operator is leaning well over the patient to increase the compression force and therefore the effectiveness of the technique. As the right hand pushes back on the anterior superior iliac spine, the left hand is pushing forwards on the ischial tuberosity and the operator is rocking from his left leg to his right to maximise the forces at the sacro-iliac joint.

Prone sacro-iliac thrust backwards alternative hold (1)

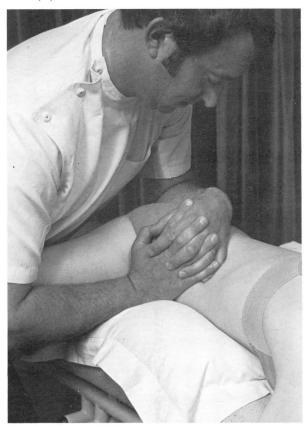

This alternative hold shows the operator's hands interlaced which some operators find more comfortable and effective.

Prone sacro-iliac thrust backwards alternative hold (2)

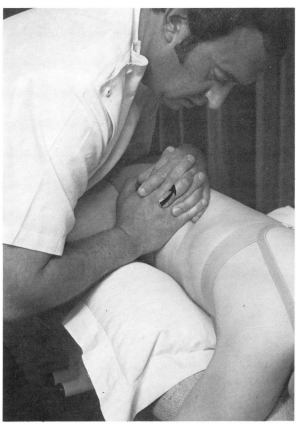

This shows the previous hold with the technique fully applied. Note that the operator has rotated his own shoulders to the left, thereby flexing the patient's hip further and is therefore forcing the ilium backwards.

137

Prone sacro-iliac articulation and thrust

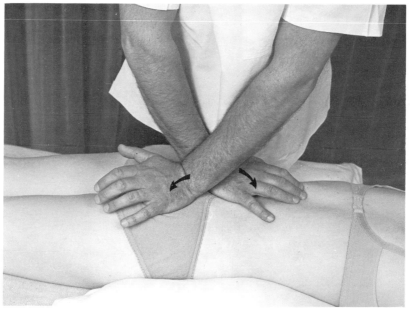

A similar "cross hands" technique to that used for a posterior innominate can be used for an anterior. The difference here is that the operator is holding the sacrum in towards the lumbar spine, and the other hand is thrusting over the posterior inferior iliac spine to encourage movement in a backwards direction. This is a somewhat inefficient leverage, but will sometimes be useful.

Supine thrust backwards on sacro-iliac (1)

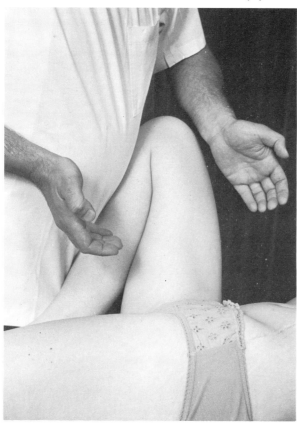

Using basically similar holds to the technique shown in the prone position, the same lesion can be treated in a supine position. The patient's hip is abducted and flexed and the operator is about to reach under the ischial tuberosity with his right hand and about to press backwards on the anterior superior iliac spine with the left hand.

Supine thrust backwards on sacro-iliac backwards (2)

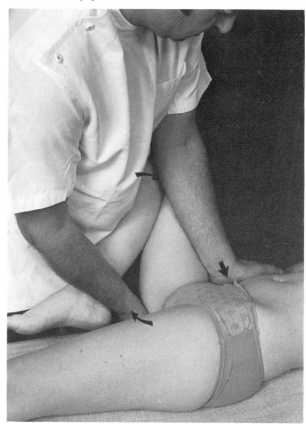

In this picture hands are applied and the operator has used his left forearm to further abduct the patient's hip. He is rocking from the patient's feet towards her head. If the pull on the ischial tuberosity is maintained, and the pressure on the anterior spine is increased, the ilium will be rocked backwards.

Sitting sacro-iliac thrust backwards

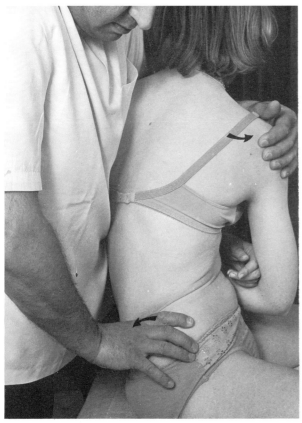

This technique for an anterior innominate relies on the operator developing a small oscillating movement with the patient's trunk and then applying a force on the ilium to break fixation in a backwards direction. Note that the patient is seated astride a narrow table to help stabilise the pelvis. Small degrees of side-bending to the side of lesion will help localise the leverages to the desired point.

Supine sacro-iliac thrust backwards (1)

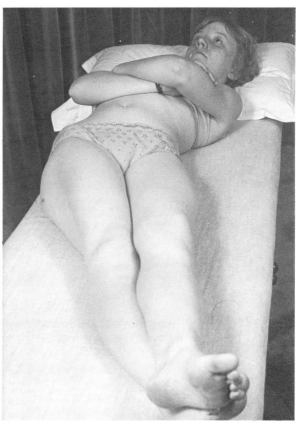

This technique is often called the "Chicago" technique as it originated from the Chicago school of Osteopathy. Note that in the preliminary positioning the patient is side-bent to one side and that the legs are crossed in such a way that the spine is beginning to rotate to the other side. There are various different hand and arm positions, but the folded arm position is being used here as most patients find it comfortable.

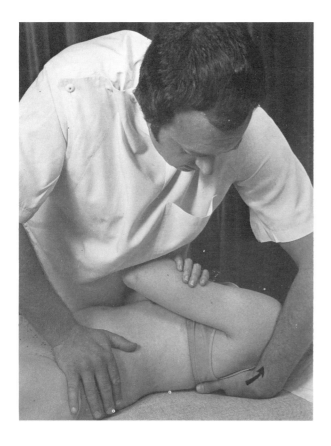

Supine sacro-iliac thrust backwards (2)

The holds are applied here with the operator pressing backwards on the anterior superior iliac spine and clasping the patient's scapula in preparation to rotate the patient's spine towards himself. A vital factor here is the maintenance of side-bending away from the operator to keep the lower lumbar tissues from excessive strain, and to make the technique more effective.

139

Supine sacro-iliac thrust backwards (3)

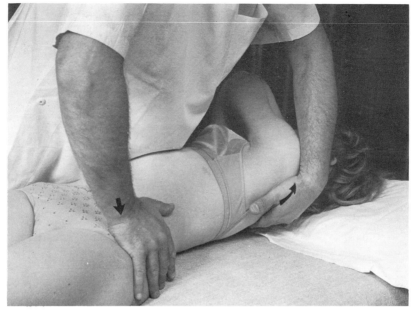

Note in this picture that the operator has placed the patient's hands behind her own neck. This sometimes helps to stabilise the levers, although most patients find this less comfortable.

Supine sacro-iliac thrust backwards (4)

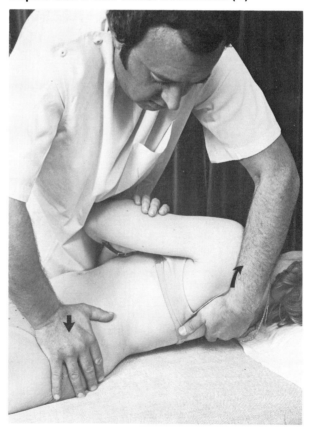

This shows a modification of the previous technique where the operator is pushing as much towards himself as towards the table. This will have the effect of localising the force more to the lumbo-sacral facet on that side as to the sacro-iliac joint. The patient's hip is kept in contact with the table at all times and if this pressure is made fairly firm the effect of this compression will minimise the amount of rotation necessary with the upper hand.

Supine sacro-iliac thrust (5)

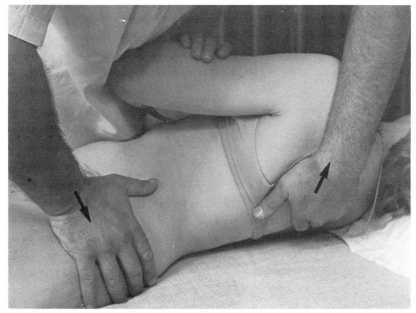

This closer view shows more clearly the direction of force for the lumbo-sacral joint.

Supine leg tug (1)

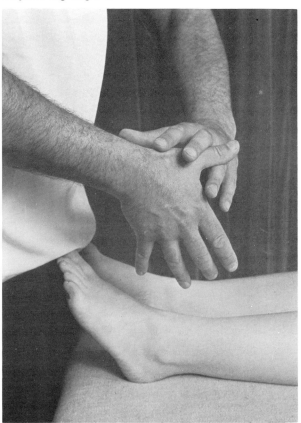

In many cases of sacro-iliac dysfunction there is an upwards element in the fixation as well as a forward or backward one. This is one way of applying a hold to the ankle to form a comfortable grip which will tighten as a pull is applied and will not dig in, or pull the skin too much.

Supine leg tug (2)

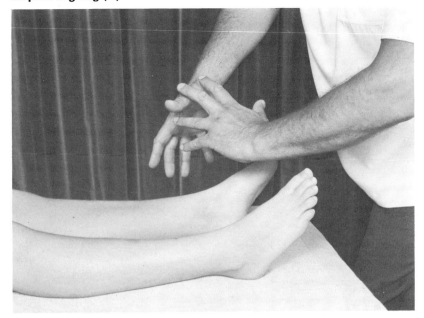

The view from the other side is shown here to aid clarity.

Supine leg tug (3)

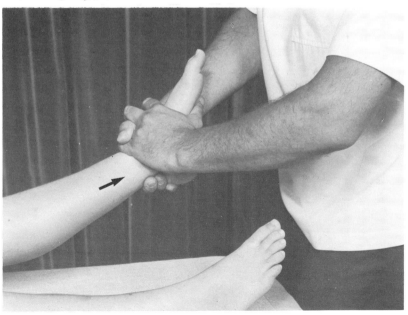

The completed hold is shown here from one side, the complete technique description is given in the next picture caption.

Supine leg tug (4)

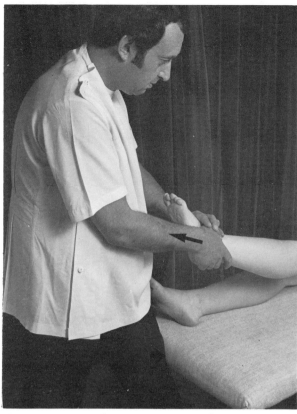

This shows the hold applied, adduction introduced to stabilise the hip and leg, flexion applied to place the hip in a neutral position, and slight internal rotation applied as well. The operator has turned his body slightly to one side, and has stabilised his leg against the table. The key to efficient leg tug techniques is to apply tension and maintain it while applying a further force, rather than using the leg as a "whip".

Side-lying sacro-iliac articulation backwards

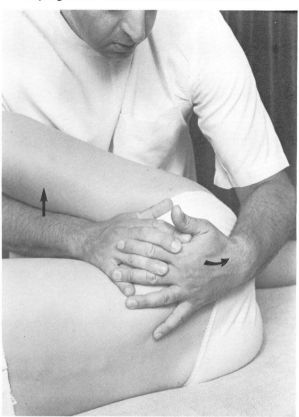

This hold can be used to articulate the ilium in a backward direction. Different amounts of abduction of the hip will alter the part of the joint affected.

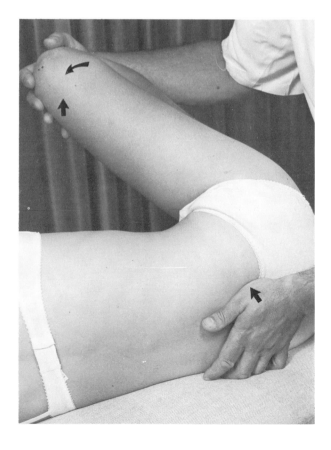

Mobilising sacro-iliac backwards

This hold, where the operator is holding back on the sacrum, is useful for mobilising the ilium in a backward direction. Once again, different degrees of abduction of the hip, and varying amounts of rotation will optimise the force.

Section H
Techniques for the lumbar area

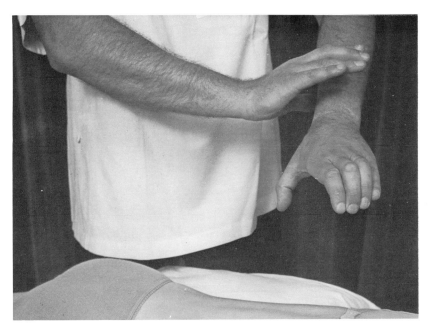

Side-shifting test and articulation (1)

This shows the basic hand hold to be applied for rocking the lumbar spine into a side-shifting direction. The first finger and thumb of the operator are to be applied to the transverse processes of one of the lumbar vertebrae.

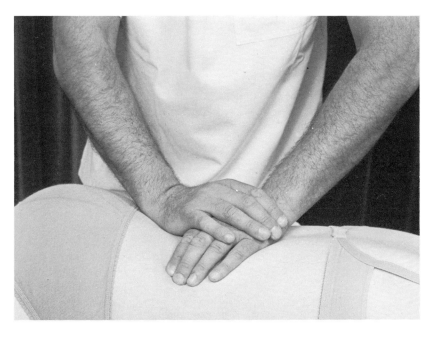

Side-shifting test and articulation (2)

The hands are applied and the operator has side-shifted the lumbar spine by using the reinforced thumbs to push on the transverse process of the affected vertebra. Note that this is a dynamic technique and that the position is not held for any period but is oscillated from side to side to the position shown in the next picture.

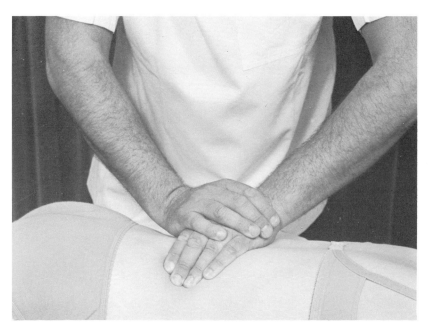

Side-shifting test and articulation (3)

This shows the alternate position to the previous picture in that the hands are pulling the vetebra towards the operator. Note that as far as possible, this is a true side-shift rather than a side-bending action. The operator's elbows are held away from the sides to allow the widest spread of downward pressure and therefore avoid excess discomfort for the patient.

Lumbar traction

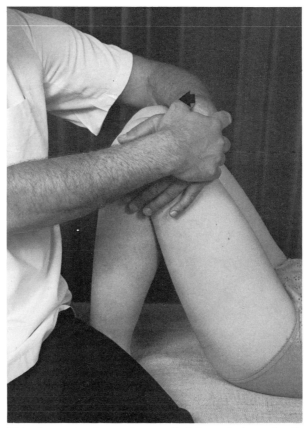

This shows simple traction applied through the patient's flexed hips. The operator is stabilising the patient's feet by lightly fixing them with his own thigh. Despite the seeming simplicity of this hold, quite strong traction can be applied merely by leaning back.

Lumbar flexion

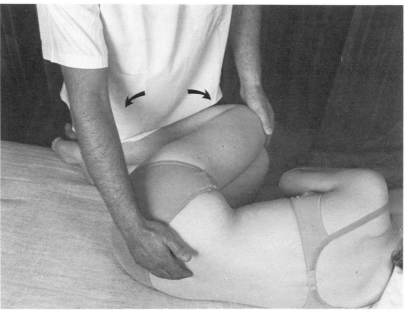

This shows one of the basic holds for applying lumbar flexion. Note that the operator has placed the patient in a stable position in the middle of the table and has got the patient's flexed legs comfortably resting on his abdomen. In this case the operator's left hand is guiding the knees into flexion while the other hand is merely palpating the interspaces for relative ranges of movement.

Strong lumbar flexion

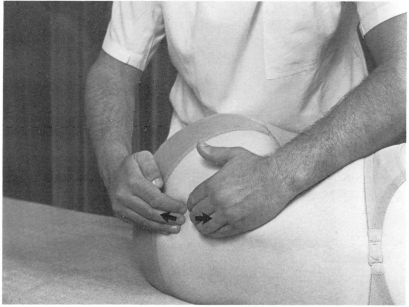

In this hold, the operator is fixing the patient's flexed legs on his abdomen, and using both hands to work on the spine. The left hand is holding back on the upper of the two vertebrae and the right hand is pulling the lower vertebra further into flexion. Subtle degrees of side-bending can be introduced, as can rotation because the operator has induced a fair degree of compression, thereby maximising the effect of any small movement later applied.

Sacral hold for lumbar flexion (1)

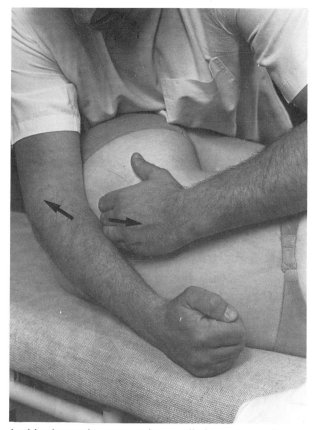

In this picture the operator has applied very strong flexion by a combination of extreme flexion of the patient's hips, a very strong hold with the right forearm, and a firm pull with the left hand on one spinous process. Once again, due to the amount of compression applied, the slightest degree of side-bending or rotation induced will have a marked effect. Although the operator is bent over, a lot of strain is reduced as he is resting partly on the patient's left hip, which also helps to stabilise the technique.

Sacral hold for lumbar flexion from the back (2)

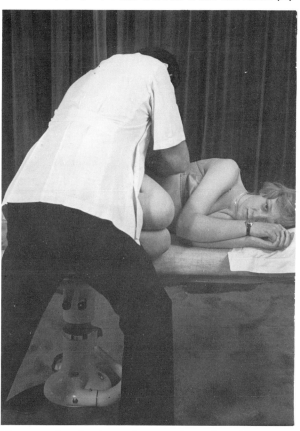

The rear view is shown here to show the wide stance necessary to produce stability when applying the techniques of flexion etc.

Lumbar flexion in side-bending

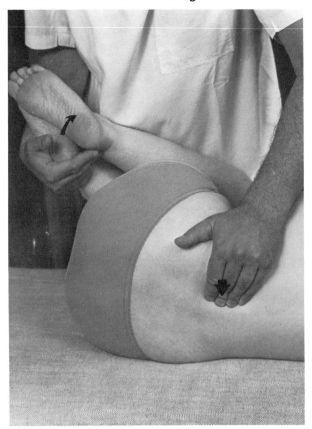

Here flexion with side-bending is being applied to the lumbar spine. The operator's left hand is pushing down carefully on the lateral side of the spinous processes. This technique can be made considerably stronger by the operator slipping his right hand through and applying it to the lateral side of the patient's left thigh.

Lumbar flexion in side-bending

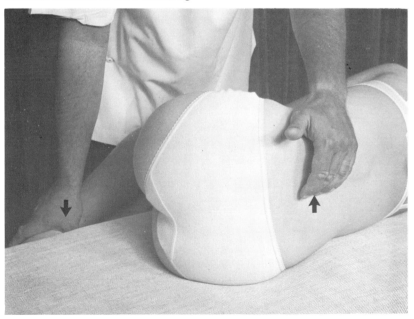

Side-bending towards the table can be induced with this hold. It requires more effort on behalf of the operator than the previous one shown, but is sometimes useful.

Lumbar extension articulation

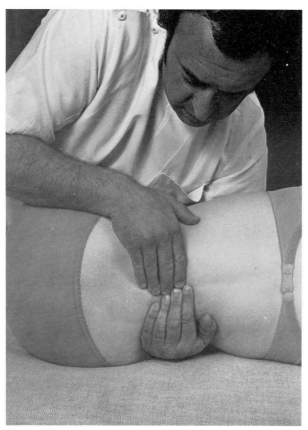

In this hold the operator has reached under the patient and has clasped over the lamina of the vertebra being worked. The other hand reinforces this hold and the patient's flexed knees are being pushed towards the patient's pelvis. This counter-pressure will induce extension at the lumbar spine. Varied degrees of rotation and side-bending can be brought into play as well.

Lumbar extension articulation alternative hold

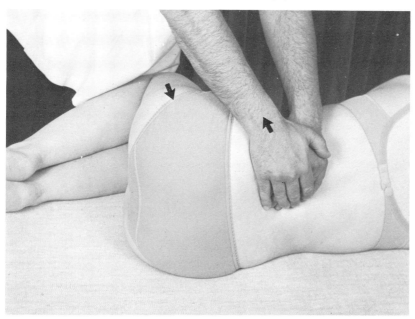

Here is shown an alternative hold for inducing extension in the lumbar and dorso-lumbar area. This has the advantage that the operator does not have to slide his own hand under the patient, but has the disadvantage that the technique is not so strong or so localised. Note that the operator is minimising the strain on one hand by overlaying it with the other.

Supine flexion and side-bending articulation

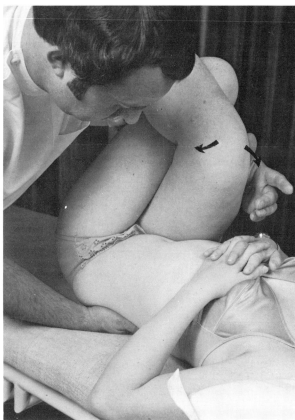

Supine flexion

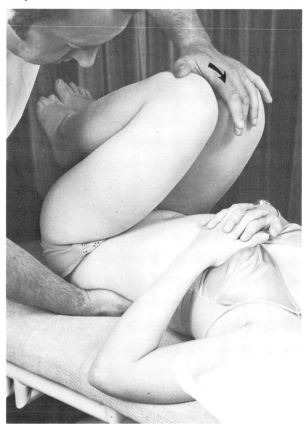

In this supine hold the operator has crossed the patient's legs to induce a degree of side-bending, and has threaded his hand behind the knees to induce flexion. The underneath hand is fixing on one or several spinous or transverse processes. The operator can then produce oscillatory side-bending, combined with varying degrees of flexion. This technique requires the patient to have unhampered hip movement. This would seem to be very hard work, but provided the patient's hips are flexed beyond 90 degrees the force necessary to maintain the thighs in this position need not be very great unless the patient is of an exceptionally heavy build.

A simpler hold than the previous one suitable for light subjects is shown here. This is most suitable in children and where large degrees of side-bending are not considered necessary. The underneath hand can perform various functions. It can hold back on a transverse or spinous process, it can push or pull laterally or vertically on them as well.

Side-lying soft tissue kneading

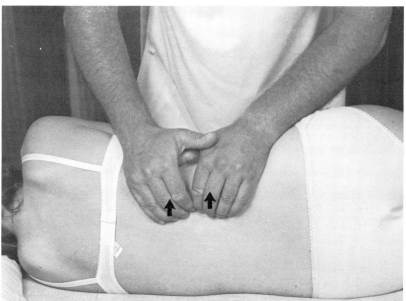

Side-lying soft-tissue stretching can be performed with the fingertips in this way. The widest possible spread of fingers produces the least discomfort, and is the least strain on the operator.

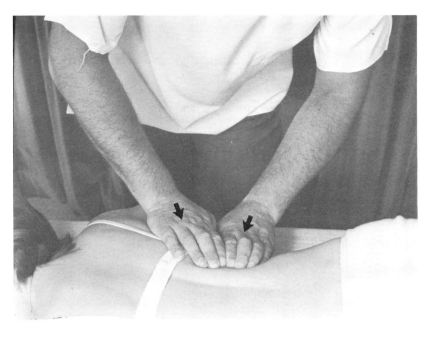

Prone soft tissue cross-fibre kneading

Soft-tissue kneading towards the spine is sometimes useful, particularly in very heavily muscled types, or where access to the other side is difficult as in a domiciliary situation. This widespread finger pressure can be used.

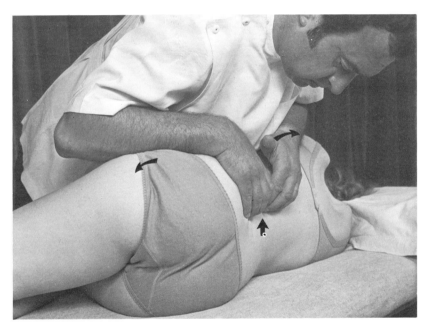

Side-lying side-bending with other components (1)

This position allows the operator to perform strong side-bending, and vary the force of the technique by applying a pull through the upper or the lower component of the combined lever system by pushing more or less firmly with either arm. The fingertips are hooked around the spinous processes and the operator is leaning on his forearms to induce a degree of compression to stabilise the levers.

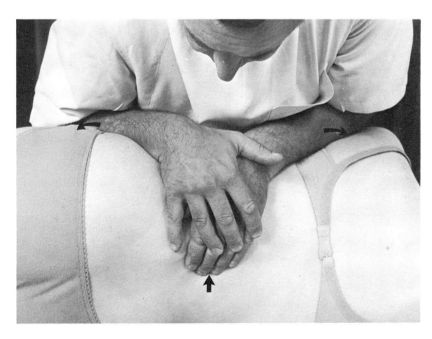

Side-lying side-bending with other components (2)

This shows another view of the previous technique with the one difference that the operator has induced a degree of backward rotation in the pelvis by placing his forearm in front of the patient's anterior superior iliac spine and is pushing backwards at the same time as the induction of side-bending. This serves to strengthen the technique without applying any greater force as the operator has brought another component of direction into the technique. Compression is available merely by leaning on the forearms.

153

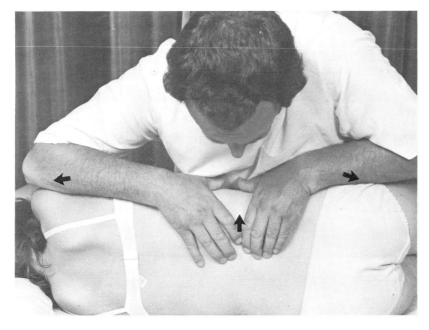

Foraminal gapping

In this hold the operator is inducing straight side-bending. If this is maintained for some time a "foraminal gapping" force is applied, which is useful in nerve root entrapment syndromes.

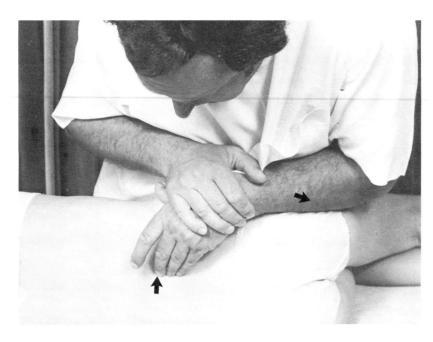

Foraminal gapping

This "foraminal gapping" hold utilises body weight rather than muscle power. The operator is pulling up under the spinous processes, and leaning on the ilium to locally side-bend the spine.

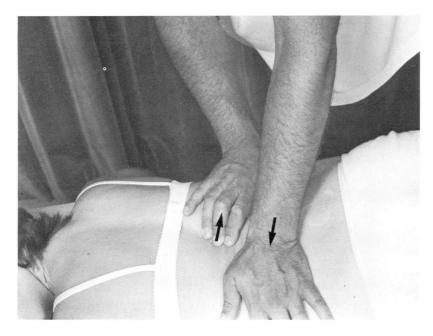

Specific push and pull on spine

This hold can be used for "push and pull". The hands are applying force in opposing directions. The left is applied to the transverse processes, and the right to the spinous processes to produce a strong rotory force to a specific segment.

Push and pull on spinous processes

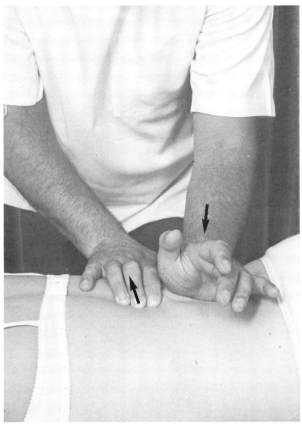

In this hold the push and pull is applied to the spinous processes.

Direct spinous process springing

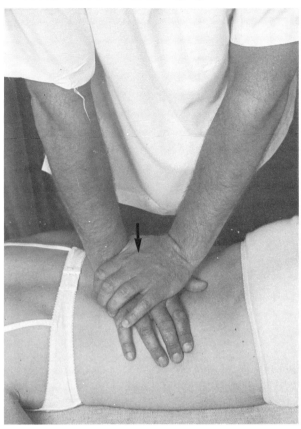

Direct springing in an antero-posterior direction is shown here. This must always be a carefully graduated force so as not to adversely irritate the coeliac plexus. It is most useful when gently oscillated over the dorso-lumbar region where the facet planes allow least movement in that direction.

Specific segmental articulation (1)

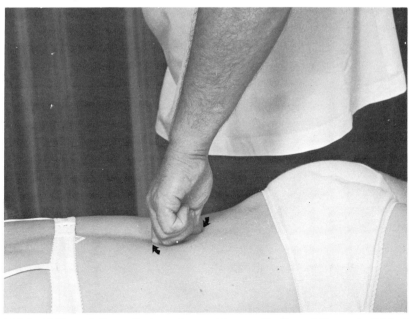

This hold, if carefully applied, can be used to specifically mobilise an individual segment. It can be used virtually throughout the spine, and if carefully applied, is not uncomfortable.

155

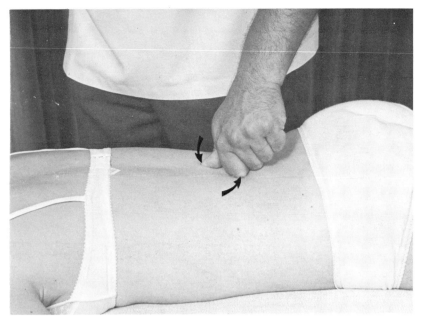

Specific segmental articulation (2)

This shows the opposite rotation movement to the previous picture.

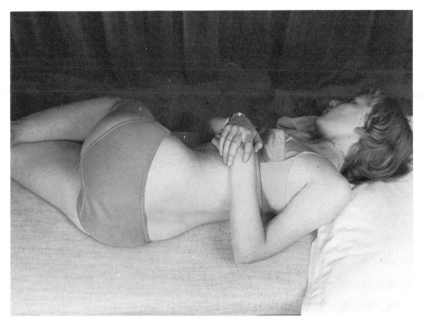

Combined leverage and thrust position (1)

This shows the basic preliminary position for the application of a combined leverage and thrust technique in the lumbar spine. Note that the patient is placed in such a position on the table that the upper knee is just over the edge.The lower shoulder has been taken through in one of various ways until it is lying anterior to the patient's pelvis. The lower scapula has been protracted from the chest wall slightly to allow further thoracic rotation if necessary without inducing discomfort. The upper leg is flexed at the hip and the patient's foot is comfortably hooked behind the other knee so that the pelvis is allowed to rotate forwards at an angle of approximately 20 degrees. As this is a somewhat torsioned position it is not comfortable to hold it for long.

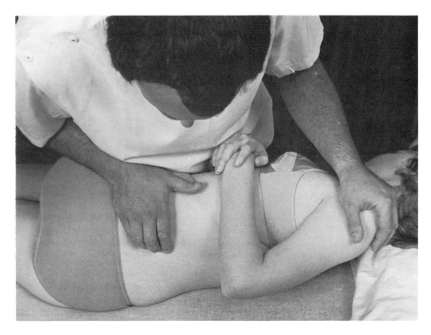

Combined leverage and thrust (2)

Here the hands are applied just preliminary to the thrust. The patient, in this case has been asked to clasp her own wrist to stabilise the shoulder girdle. The operator has applied his thrusting arm (right) to the sulcus between gluteus medius and gluteus maximus. He has hooked his fingers round the underside of the vertebra to which he is going to thrust. The thrusting arm is kept well into the side, and the elbow is behind the midline of the body. The stabilising hand is applied to the anterior surface of the patient's shoulder avoiding excess pressure over the long head of biceps. The whole patient can be rolled back and forth until the optimum tension is sensed at the contact point. The thrust can then be applied as a rapid movement towards the table with the operator's right arm.

Alternative hold combined leverage and thrust (3)

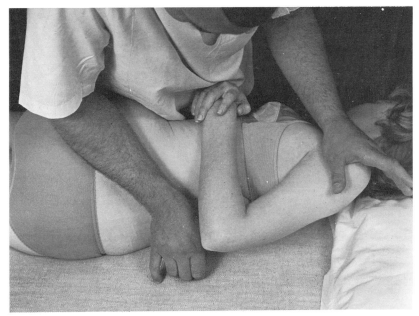

In this alternative hold for the combined leverage and thrust, the operator has a somewhat stronger lever available. This hold however has the disadvantage that the operator does not have as accurate a sense of tension as the hand is not actually applied to the vertebra in question.

Alternative hold combined leverage and thrust (4)

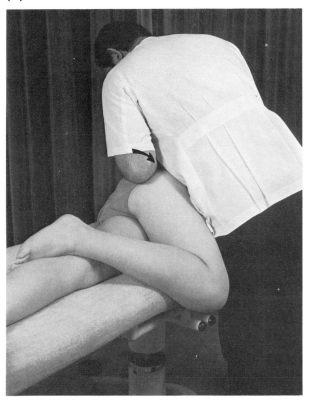

The rear view is shown here to emphasise the importance of correct operator posture. Note that the operator has the front of his thighs applied to the edge of the table, the leg on the thrusting side is placed behind the other leg to lock his own spine in rotation and extension and that the thrusting elbow is behind the midline of the body. His own thigh is resting against that of the patient to add stability when rolling the patient back and forth. The patient's knee is clear of the edge of the table so that rotation can be applied if necessary and without hindrance. The table height is such that the operator does not have to stand on tip-toes, or bend his knees excessively to make satis-factory contact.

Alternative hold combined leverage and thrust (5)

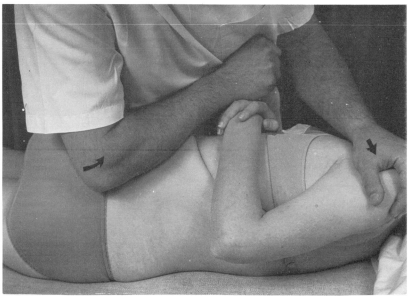

Another variation of the basic hold is shown here. The operator is using the inner side of the thrusting forearm applied to the posterior superior iliac spine and the crest of the ilium. This allows extension to be applied more easily than the previous method and can be modified to produce a forward rotational force on the ilium. Although very strong, this method also has the disadvantage of not allowing contact to be made with the lesion point at the moment of thrust.

Alternative hold combined leverage and thrust (6)

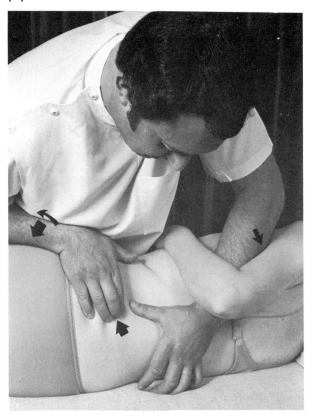

In this commonly used hold the operator has threaded his left forearm through between the patient's side and her own arm. This has the advantage that it allows the upper hand to take part in the technique by fixing on the affected segment, but it has the severe disadvantage that the operator has to dissipate a high proportion of his weight towards the upper lever which should only be a stabiliser for the lower component. There is also the danger of applying too much force to the shoulder and damaging it or the upper ribs. Notwithstanding this, this can be a very useful hold if used with care.

Alternative hold combined leverage and thrust (7)

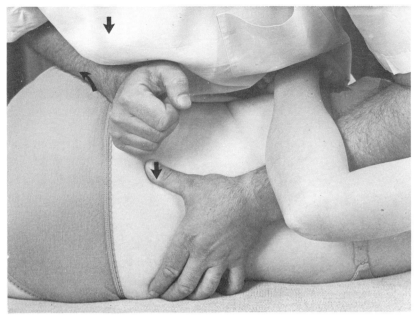

This alternative view shows the operator's thrusting hand applied further laterally, so that the body can be used to reinforce the thrust on the forearm.

Alternative hold combined leverage and thrust (8)

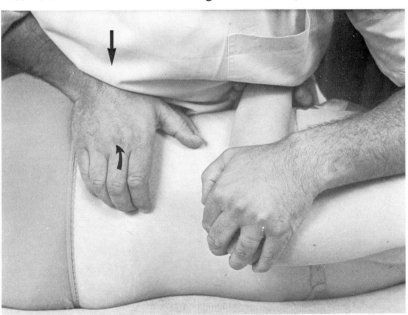

This hold combines the last two methods, in that, the operator is holding the patient's upper arm with his left forearm. This allows the operator to slightly vary several aspects of the technique. Extension and side-bending can be brought into play with only very subtle movements.

Alternative hold combined leverage and thrust (9)

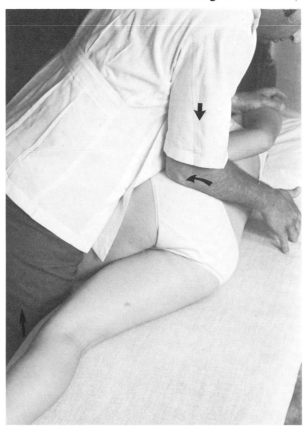

This hold for applying a thrust to the lumbar spine is very strong. Note that the operator has stepped over the patient's leg and is flexing it between his own legs. This allows much stronger flexion forces to be used than with the leg on the table, if this is deemed necessary.

Alternative hold combined leverage and thrust (10)

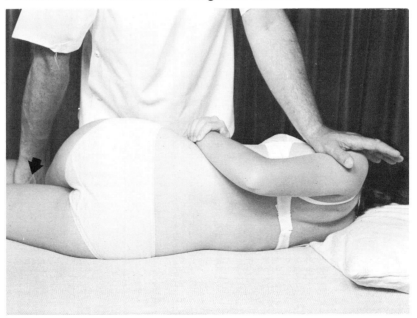

Some operators find this hold useful for applying lumbar thrusts. The disadvantages of not having a finger on the segment concerned are obvious, however, with practice, accuracy can be achieved.

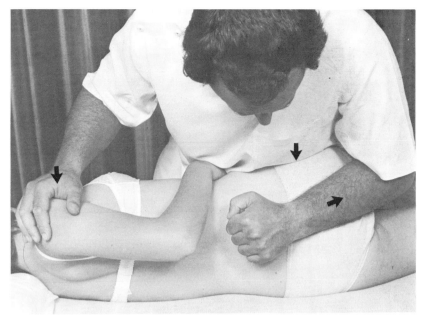

Sacral thrust

The hold shown here is applicable to direct sacral thrusts. The operator is maintaining firm compression on the pelvis and is then using a very rapid thrust into flexion on the sacrum. If the force is rapid enough, most of the effect will be on the lumbo-sacral facets rather than anywhere else.

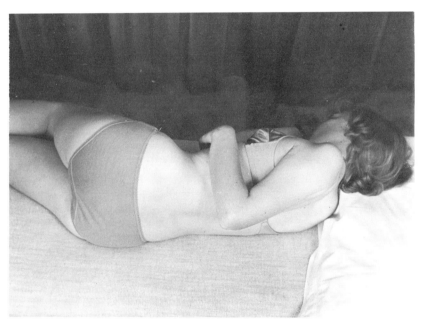

Minimal leverage thrust (1)

This is the basic position for applying a minimal leverage thrust to the lumbar spine. A careful comparison with this and the position for the combined leverage and thrust shown earlier will reveal many subtle changes. The patient's upper leg is just placed comfortably in front of the lower leg. The shoulders are almost perpendicular to one another. The patient is in a non-torsioned position, and is completely relaxed.

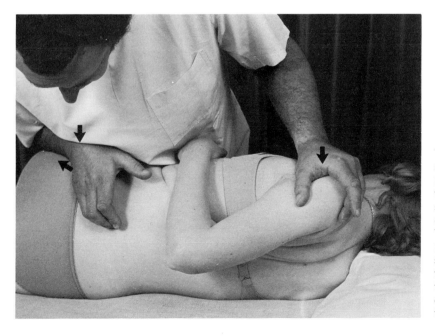

Minimal leverage thrust (2)

The minimal lever technique has been started here. Note that the patient has not been placed in any great degree of torsion, the operator has applied considerable compression via the application of his own chest to his forearm. The operator's upper hand has applied a pressure down towards the table to stabilise the levers. The direction of thrust in this particular case is down towards the table and then along the crest of the ilium to "gap" the upper facet of the affected vertebra.

161

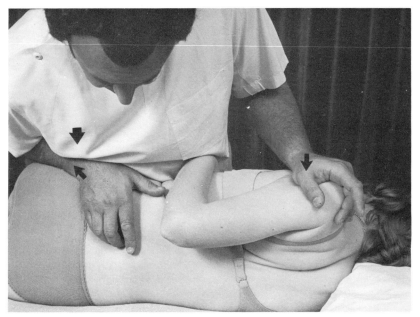

Minimal leverage thrust (3)

The minimal leverage thrust has been completed here. The final position will be seen to be very little different from the commencing position. Slightly more rotation is evident, and the operator's body is seen to be slightly lower towards the table as further compression has been applied. The use of compression here minimises the quantity of all the other levers necessary. The whole point of minimal lever techniques is that the patient could be taken into any of the lever directions further than they are at the completion of the technique. The combination of all the directions, plus the compression and very high speed completes the technique.

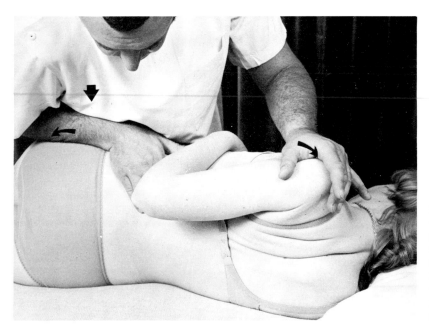

Minimal leverage thrust in side-bending

In this picture, the operator is using a minimal leverage technique, emphasising side-bending and extension. Note that although the patient is obviously in side-bending, it is very slight as the compression force is focusing the forces. The whole point of minimal leverage techniques is not their use without a lever, but the use of as minimal a lever as possible in the circumstances.

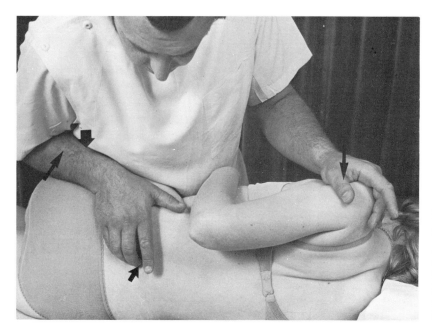

Minimal leverage thrust using compression

In this minimal leverage approach the operator is using rotation emphasised with flexion. Once again the degree of total movement is very small but the effect of compression has localised the force.

Lumbar contra-rotation in opposite direction to usual

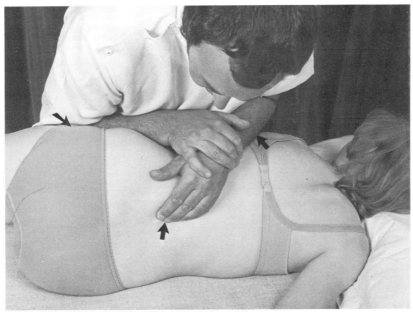

This hold is another of contra-rotation, except that the pelvis is being rotated backwards and the shoulder forwards. This type of approach sometimes allows breaking of fixation where the conventional direction has not achieved full flexibility. It is most appropriate for the dorso-lumbar area, and can be used as a combined lever approach or a minimal lever approach. Whereas in the usual lumbar technique, the operator thrusts on the lower component, and stabilises the upper component; in this technique the opposite is true. The upper component is pulled into rotation towards the operator, aided by the fingers pulling upwards on the spinous processes. The operator is pushing backwards on the anterior superior iliac spine with his other forearm.

Lumbar adjustive traction

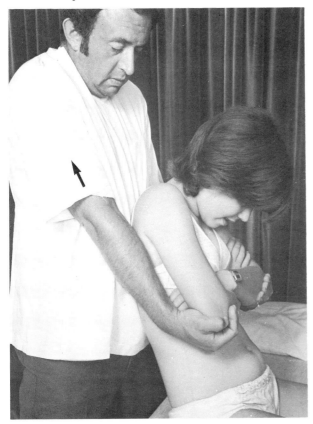

This hold can be used for applying a direct traction force to the lumbar spine. Varying degrees of side-bending and rotation can be used, and then a sharp lift will localise the force to the segment desired.

Standing traction (1)

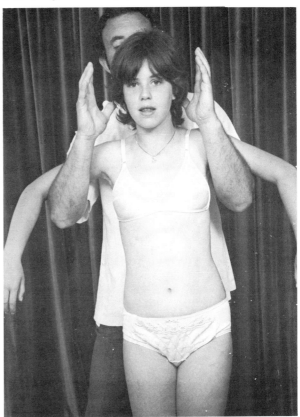

In young people a traction side-bending force can be useful, particularly in cases of scoliosis. This hold can be used for this purpose. Most of the weight is taken by the patient's shoulders, but the hands lock under the mastoid processes to assist.

163

Standing traction (2)

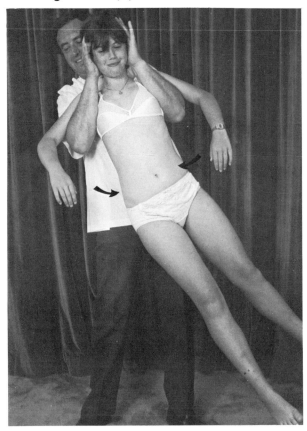

The hold has been taken up, the patient lifted, and a side-bending force applied. The pendulum action is emphasised in the direction necessary.

Prone dorso-lumbar thrust

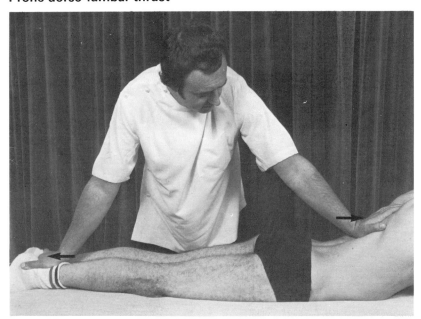

This position can be used for oscillatory pressure on the dorso-lumbar area to encourage extension. The patient is resting on his bent elbows. Rotation can be introduced by emphasising the pressure on one side of the spine on the transverse processes. Side-bending can also be brought in by pushing the transverse processes towards the head on one side. To turn this technique into a thrust technique it is necessary to set up a slow oscillation and at the end of one of the ranges of movement, applying a thrust to the spinous, or transverse processes as necessary. This can be a very uncomfortable process if excess force is used or if the area is very sensitive as in osteochondrosis, or osteoporosis.

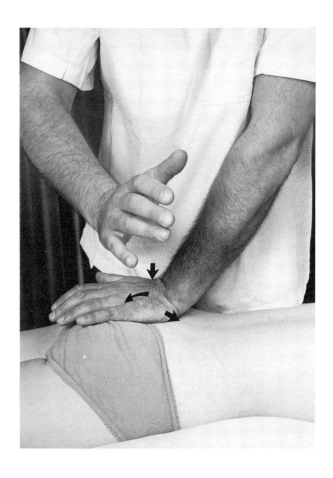

Prone lumbo-sacral thrust

Although this basic hold is more usually used for mobilising the sacro-iliac joints, it can be used for causing a gapping at the lumbo-sacral facets. The operator has applied firm pressure towards the table, then towards the patient's head and lastly into flexion of the sacrum by pushing with a rocking motion towards the patient's feet with a fairly sharp thrust.

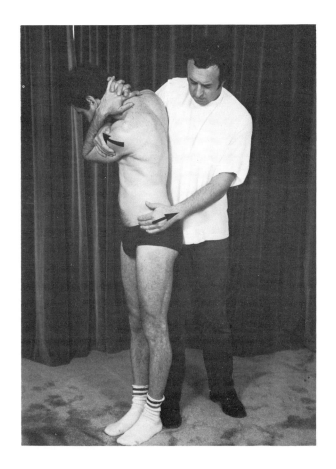

Standing lumbo-sacral thrust

This shows a technique which is fairly unusual, and yet can be very useful. The basic principles of any thrust techniques are being used, namely rotation to one side and side-bending to the other with varying amounts of flexion or extension. The added benefit of the standing position is that the operator can induce some degree of traction if necessary. The contra-rotation here is obviously in a direction where the pelvis is moving backwards. Greater degrees of side-bending or rotation can be induced by placing one leg in front of the other. The thrust comes from the upper component aided by a sharp pull backwards on the pelvis.

165

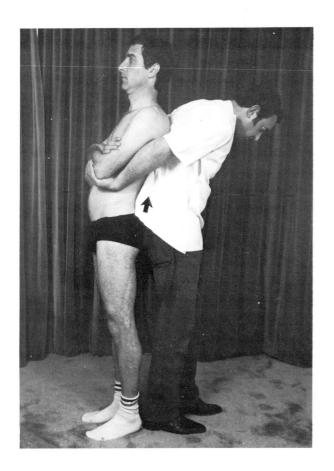

Vertical adjustment (1)

The use of a vertical component in lumbar techniques is very helpful, particularly where there is a disc herniation complicating the lesion picture. This hold allows the operator to lift the patient without too much effort providing he is at least the same height as the patient. Much of the patient's weight is taken on the operator's sacrum.

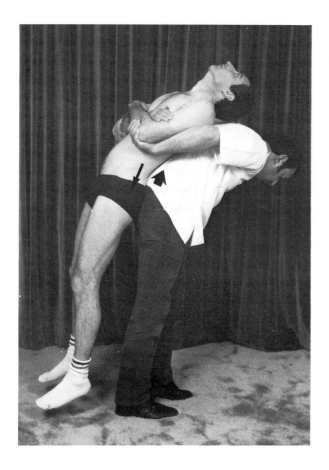

Vertical adjustment (2)

The patient has been lifted and asked to extend his head to place the whole spine in extension. The thrust is performed, not by lifting the patient, more by coming up on the balls of the feet then rapidly dropping onto the heels, thereby applying a rapid traction force to the lumbar spine. Varying degrees of side-bending and rotation can be applied by altering the hold slightly to focus the force at a particular segment. Note this technique is not to be applied if the patient has difficulty in extending beyond the straight line as it will induce intense discomfort.

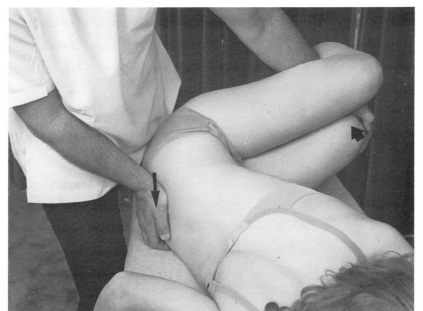

'Two-man' technique (1)

Several techniques have been evolved which require the use of two, or more operators, or an operator and one or more assistants. This shows the main operator's hold for a two man technique for thrusting, or applying very strong articulation to the lumbar spine. The patient is placed in a semi-simms position and the operator is pulling up on the patient's knees (assisted in lifting them by the second operator if necessary). The patient's hips are maintained in a flexed position beyond 90 degrees. The amount of flexion being varied according to which part of the lumbar spine is being worked. The operator is resting the knee nearer the patient's feet on the table to get as close as possible. The right hand is firmly pushing towards the table on the side of the spinous processes. Once the operator has established himself in position, the second operator can take up his hold.

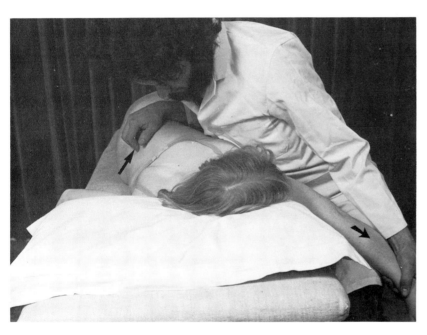

'Two-man' technique (2)

The second operator in this picture has taken up his hold. He is applying traction through the patient's left arm. He is resting his chest on the patient's shoulder to stabilise the lever. He has clasped his right hand round the spinous processes of the lumbar spine above where the main operator is to clasp.

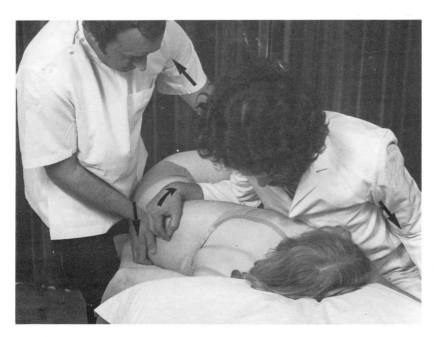

'Two-man' technique (3)

In this picture both the operators have taken up their positions. At a command from the main operator, the second operator holds his lever firmly and the main operator rotates the lower component to the left.

167

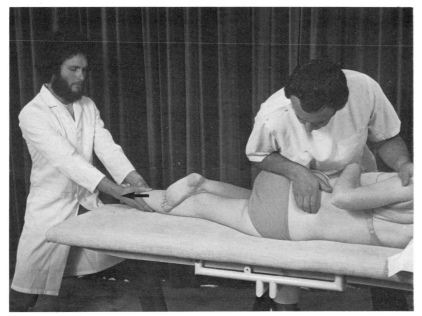

Leg traction 'two-man' technique

In this technique the main operator takes up a position as he would normally to perform a thrust to the lumbar spine. The second operator applies traction on the lower leg and very often the main operator can then get the lumbar spine in a more optimum position for the thrust. This is particularly useful in cases where sciatica prevents rotation of the lumbar spine. The pull can be consistent or coincident with the lumbar thrust.

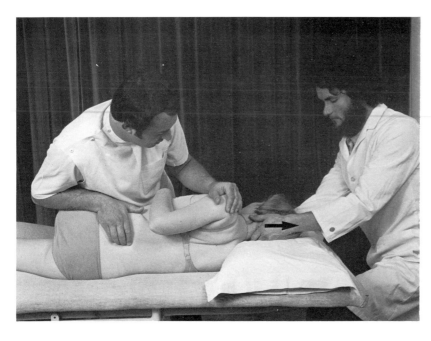

Head traction 'two-man' technique

When performing lumbar thrust technique, it is sometimes difficult to achieve the correct tension at the segment in question. This can be either due to pain, or a physical block. In some cases if the second operator applies traction via the cervical column, further rotation, if using combined lever technique, or more optimum tension, if using minimum lever technique is possible. In some cases both this method and the use of leg traction can be combined. Naturally this needs three operators. In all these techniques where more than one operator is working on the patient, practice is required to achieve the optimum tension and timing and coordination between the operators.

Section I
Miscellaneous pelvic techniques

Connective tissue separation

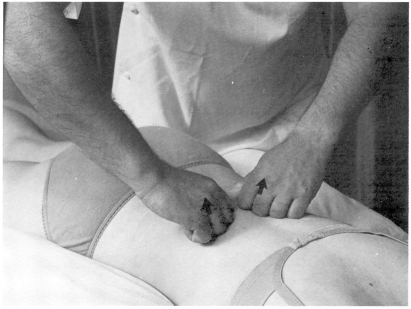

In some cases restricted flexibility can be traced back to tension in the superficial fascia and skin. This technique stretches the fascia and can actually be used to produce a cavitation and separation of the superficial tissues from the deeper ones. The operator rolls the skin between fingers and thumb to find the area of maximal resistance. He then gathers the slack and after taking it all up applies a very short sharp pull upwards to the skin. The crack that ensues sounds just like a joint sound, but in fact originates from the soft tissues.

Symphysis pubis separation

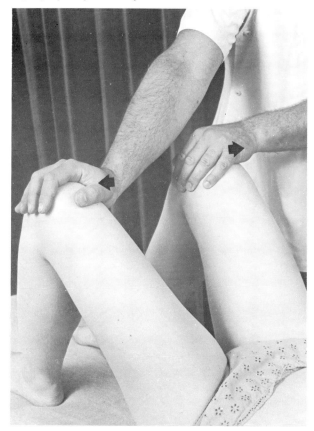

This position is used in a technique to gap the symphysis pubis. Most problems related to the symphysis pubis are due to hypermobility rather than hypomobility, and so the operator must be quite sure of the indications before applying this technique. The patient's knees and hips are flexed and the patient is asked to resist the operator's attempt to abduct the thighs, and yet allow the movement to take place a little at a time. At the optimum moment, the symphysis pubis will sometimes gap by itself. If this does not happen, the operator can apply a very short sharp thrust to the thighs in abduction.

Sacro-coccygeal joint articulation (1)

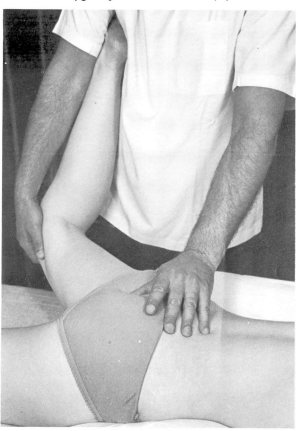

The sacro-coccygeal joint can be articulated in this position. The operator is abducting, extending and internally rotating the hip to apply tension to the tissues round the coccyx. The operator is applying his thumb to the joint to provide counter-fixation.

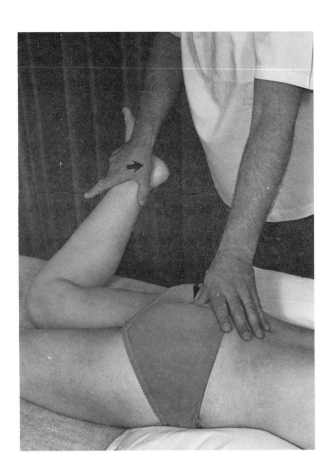

Sacro-coccygeal articulation (2)

This is a stonger leverage than the previous shown technique, except that the operator is leaving the thigh on the table to emphasise the rotation element rather than adding the abduction and extension. This position is more appropriate for dealing with tension in the more superficial tissues.

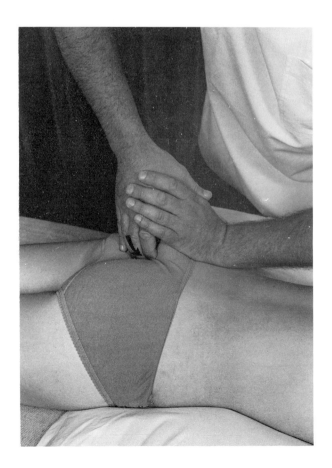

Sacro-coccygeal soft tissue kneading and stretching

Deep soft-tissue stretching can be applied with this hold. The fingers are worked in adjacent to the coccyx and then pulled laterally and upwards. This sort of technique is best held for several seconds rather than repeat too fast.

Section J
Techniques for the knee

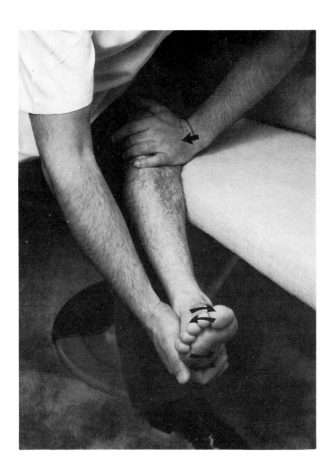

Knee articulation and meniscus thrust

This is a very useful general hold for performing several different functions in the knee. The operator has clasped the patient's femur between his own thigh and the table and has stabilised this with the palmar surface of his pronated left hand. The femur is therefore fixed. The other hand is holding the calcaneum and can produce flexion, extension, abduction, adduction, internal and external rotation as well as circumduction of the knee. This hold can be used as a general articulation or can even be used for reducing small degrees of medial, and sometimes lateral meniscus displacement. To use it for reduction of a meniscus displacement, a certain order of movement introduction is necessary. A medial meniscus usually needs abduction, external rotation, extension and then internal rotation in that order. These have to be applied with clockwise circumduction (looking towards the patient's feet). A lateral meniscus needs, strong adduction, internal rotation, extension, external rotation and counter-clockwise rotation.

Knee traction

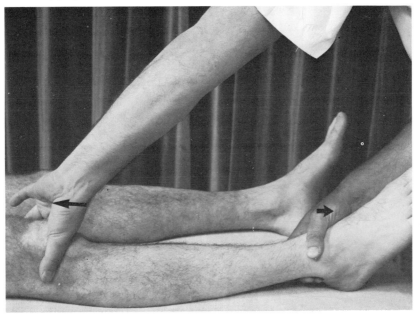

This very simple hold is useful for applying traction to the knee joint. The fact that the operator has his left hand in full pronation avoids excess pressure on the patella. The operator can use his right hand to apply traction, or different degrees of rotation in traction, as well as abduction or adduction if desired.

Postero-anterior articulation

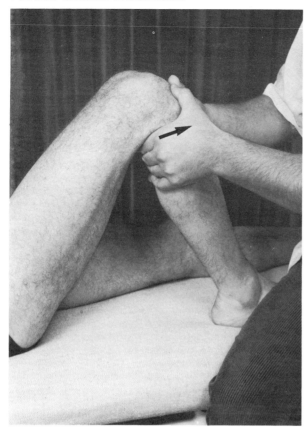

Some authorities are of the opinion that the knee can develop a lesion pattern where the tibia rides backwards on the femur. This hold can be used for correction of this situation. Note that the operator is lightly trapping the patient's foot with his own thigh to prevent the pull causing extension of the knee instead of a pure antero-posterior movement.

Antero-posterior articulation

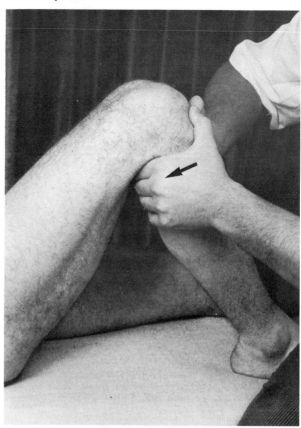

This technique is the converse of that shown in the previous picture. Note that varied degrees of rotation can be applied at the same time as the antero-posterior movement to apply the force to the medial or the lateral compartment of the knee.

Lateral shift of tibia correction (1)

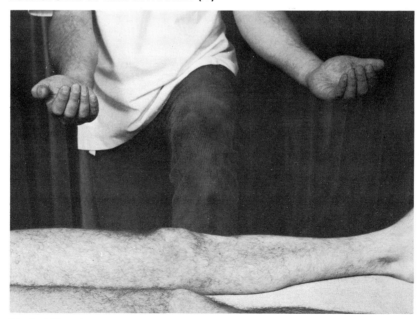

The hold here is designed to do two things. Firstly to act as a corrective force of a lateral shift of the tibia, and secondly to act as a corrective technique for small degrees of medial meniscus displacements. The left hand is about to be placed under the patient's heel. The right hand is about to be placed under the knee to clasp the lower end of the femur. The operator's knee is about to be placed on the lateral side of the tibia to drive it medially.

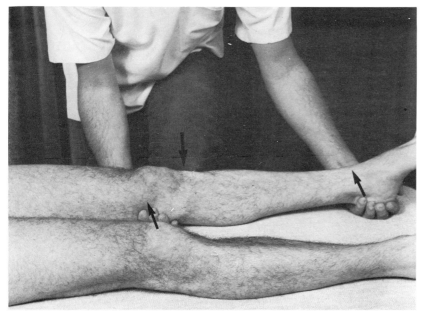

Lateral shift of tibia correction (2)

Here the hands are applied. The tibia is placed in a small degree of internal rotation so that the operator's infra-patellar tendon is placed carefully on the small plateau just below and anterior to the superior tibio-fibular joint. The operator can oscillate the knee around the axis of the applied knee. At the appropriate point of tension he pulls both hands towards himself against the fixed knee. If the patient tenses his own quadriceps at the time of the thrust, it sometimes assists the technique.

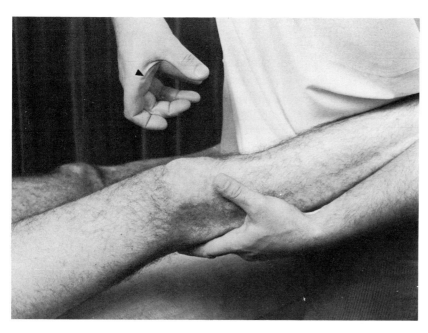

Medial shift of tibia correction (1)

One commonly used hold for applying a thrust to the knee joint is shown here. The operator is going to apply the carpo-metacarpal joint of the right hand to a variety of points on the medial side of the tibia.

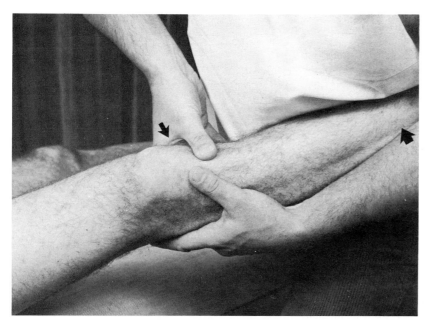

Medial shift of tibia correction (2)

The hands are applied in such a way that if the operator is clasping the leg firmly into his side, any force applied to the medial side of the knee will tend to produce a lateral gapping force. If circumduction is introduced, forces can be directed to different parts of the joint. Note that the operator has his right arm at 90 degrees to the leg to optimise any forces used. This technique will sometimes be used to deal with a situation where the tibia has moved medially, the thrust forcing it laterally. It can also be used for lateral gapping in a case of displacement of the lateral cartilage. The application of the operator's right thumb here can induce a lateral rotation element to the tibial component of the technique.

177

Lateral shift of tibia correction

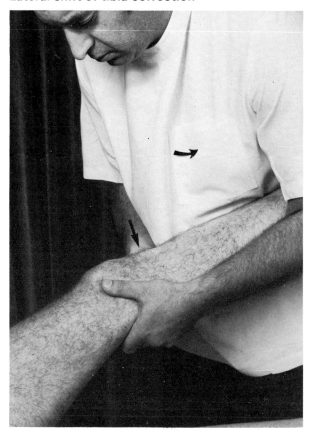

The hold shown here on the patient's left leg, is designed to be developed to deal with a situation where the tibia has moved laterally on the femur. This hold can also be used for gapping the medial side of the knee joint, with varying degrees of rotation and flexion to realign the medial meniscus. The force necessary to cause gapping in this technique is not very great providing the operator has already applied a firm pressure, and performs the thrust very sharply over a small range.

Staggered hold for tibia thrust (1)

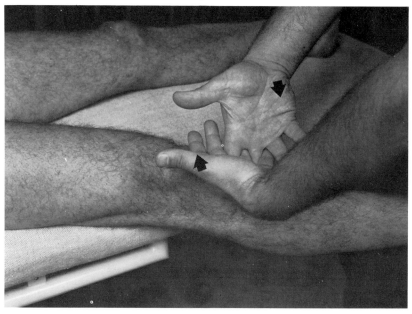

The hands are clasped in a "staggered" hold here. They are placed under the knee so that when they are firmly pushed towards each other, there will be a shearing force in the knee. The patient's foot is clasped between the operator's crossed legs just above the knees.

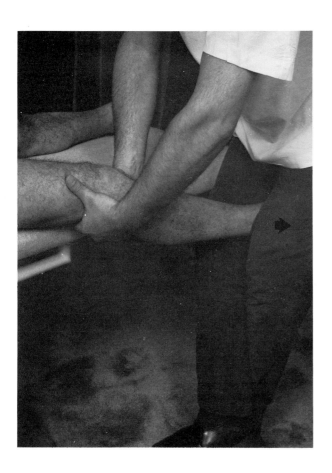

Staggered hold for tibia thrust (2)

The hold shown in the previous photo is fully applied here. As the operator circumducts the knee with the hands, he can apply the squeezing thrust with the hands and simultaneously apply traction via the crossed legs. Naturally the clasp of the hands can be varied to induce a medial force on the tibia by staggering them in the opposite way. The forces can be directed to various parts of the joint by applying the thrust at varied points of rotation and circumduction. In this way the different parts of the meniscus, medial or lateral, and the capsule can be worked. Note that the operator has his arms well abducted from his sides to increase the effect of the direction of forces.

Medial meniscus correction (1)

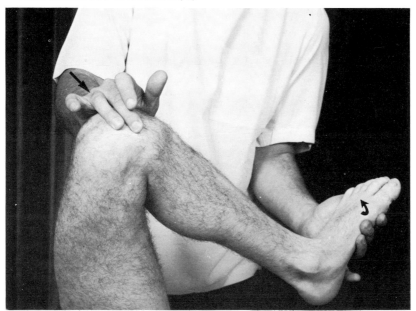

This photo is the first of a series of three. The starting point for a replacement technique for a medial meniscus displacement is shown. The knee is flexed as far as it will comfortably go. The tibia is externally rotated and the hip is adducted to gap the medial side of the knee. The technique consists of as firm a flexion as the patient can take, then a rapid extension, maintaining the medial gapping and external rotation, followed by a rapid internal rotation and holding hyperextension. To try and go through this procedure with a patient who is in great distress and pain is obviously a fraught process so the technique can be broken down into its elements and performed slowly with equal effect. As in this picture the knee is flexed and externally rotated and gently "toggled" into increased flexion. The hip is slowly rotated medially and laterally looking for the point of least tension in the knee. Extension can then slowly be introduced, while maintaining the tibial rotation and medial gapping.

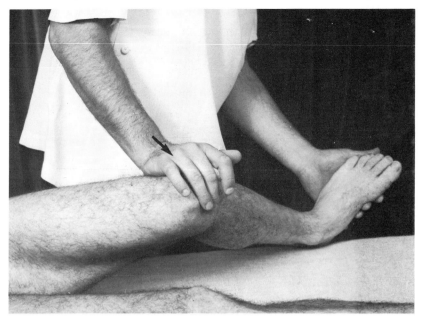

Medial meniscus correction (2)

The position here is the most critical of the sequence in this medial meniscus replacement technique. The knee is in a balanced position where the patient has "lost" control. By gently easing flexion and extension in a small range, the meniscus is allowed to relocate itself and the knee can then be eased into extension and internal rotation. Note the operator's arm tucked close into his side to utilise the rotation of the body as the prime moving force, which allows finer degrees of movement.

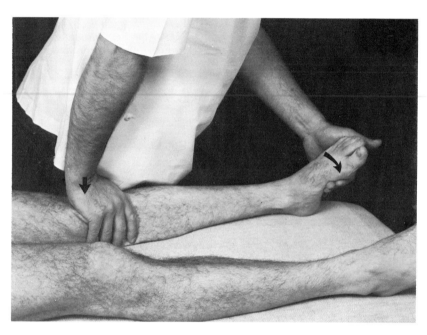

Medial meniscus correction (3)

This shows the final position of the composite technique. Note that the operator has held the knee firmly into extension using body weight. This is often necessary for several seconds as reflex spasm may pull into flexion and the meniscus is allowed to pull out again. Note also that the foot is held into internal rotation thereby helping to lock the meniscus into place.

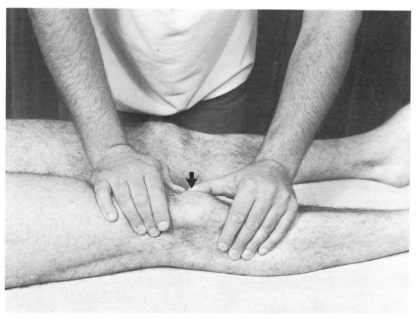

Patello-femoral articulation (1)

This simple hold is shown for articulation of the patello-femoral joint into a lateral direction of the patella. This is a useful testing procedure for provocation of a recurrent disclocation of the patella. If there is a likelihood of this, the pressure will induce an immediate protective reaction. If the technique is varied in direction, it can be used to elevate the patella and get under its edge which may be useful in conditions such as chondromalacia patellae. Note that the operator is holding back equally on the tibia and the femur to prevent rotation here, although rotation could be used if required.

Patello-femoral articulation (2)

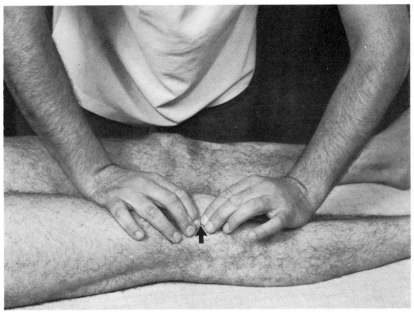

The converse of the last hold shown is being used here. This allows the operator to medially move the patella and thereby make available the lateral side of the patello-femoral joint for frictional massage etc.

Superior tibio-fibular joint gapping (1)

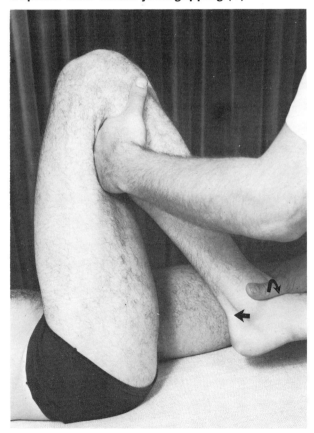

The superior tibio-fibular joint can be gapped using this hold. The operator has adducted the hip and externally rotated the tibia to get the superior aspect of the tibia to "bite" the hand. The knee is then firmly thrust into flexion and a slight exaggeration of external rotation. Note that the knee must first be tested for its ability to fully flex.

Superior tibio-fibular joint gapping (2)

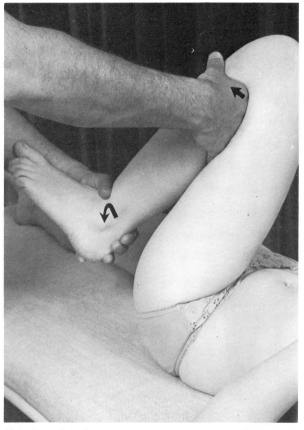

If the knee fully flexes, and the superior aspect of the fibula still does not "bite" on the thrusting hand, the operator can induce a force as in the direction of the arrow to drive the fibula forward.

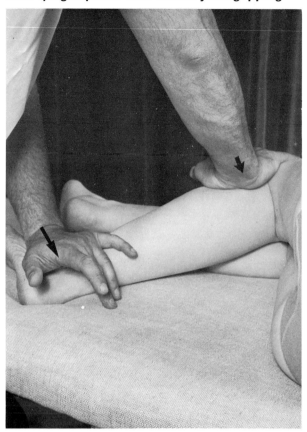

If the knee cannot fully flex, this alternative hold can be used to mobilise the superior tibio-fibular joint. The knee is placed in about 90 degrees of flexion, the foot is firmly placed on the table to induce some external rotation to bring the fibula posteriorly. The operator then applies a force to the superior aspect of the joint while maintaining the inferior part of the fibula in a stable position with the other hand. Care must be taken to avoid the lateral peroneal nerve which is very susceptible to pressure if the thrusting hand is applied carelessly.

Section K
Techniques for the foot

Tibio-taloid traction

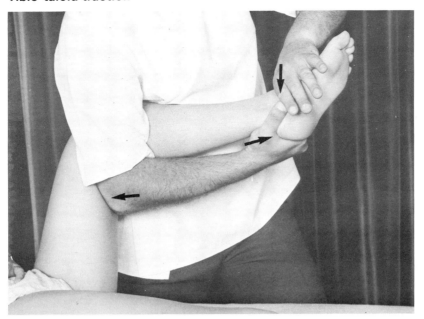

This hold can be used to gap the tibio-taloid joint. If the hands are maintained in a fixed position, and the operator then rocks from front to back, the force will be increased in a direction so as to stretch the joint. Note that the operator's right elbow is fixed against the thigh.

Tibio-taloid traction

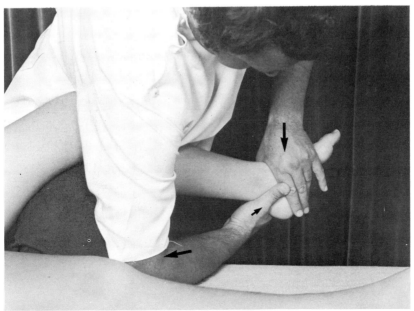

In this hold the operator has rested his right thigh on the table. The right forearm is resting on the table, and the back of the arm is pressed firmly against the inner aspect of the thigh. The right hand is kept firmly pressed against the calcaneum and then downward pressure is applied with the left hand. As two sides of the triangle formed by the thigh and the forearm and the patient's leg are maintained at the same length, a gapping force will occur at the tibio-taloid joint.

Tibio-taloid joint thrust (1)

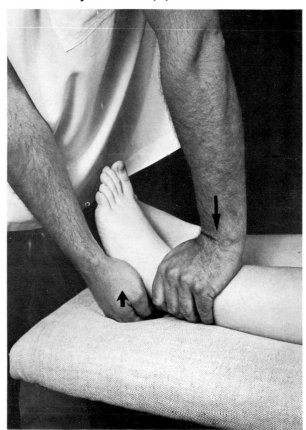

This hold can be used to drive the tibia backwards in a case where the operator has found restriction of backward gliding. Note that the right hand is holding on the calcaneum and prising it off the table. The left hand is taking up a comfortable hold on the anterior and lateral surface of the tibia, avoiding the spine of the tibia. The slack is taken out of the joint and the thrust is a very short sharp one directly backwards towards the table. Slight traction can be used via the right hand to assist the gapping force.

Tibio-taloid joint thrust (2)

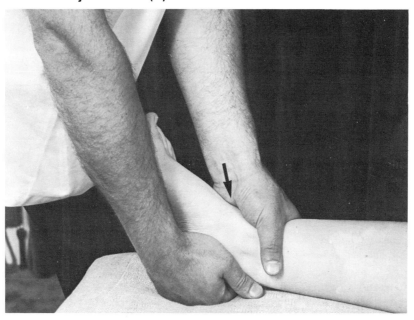

This alternative hold for driving the tibia backwards is sometimes preferable to the previous one shown as the thrusting hand is closer to the joint. Once again traction can be introduced if desired.

Tibio-taloid joint thrust (3)

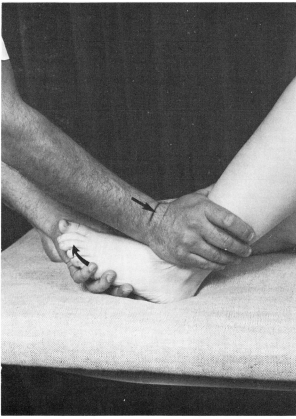

This hold is used when mobility is desired in the technique because the patient cannot relax, or if greater force is required. The ankle is alternately dorsiflexed and returned to neutral by pushing more and less firmly on the tibia, while lifting and releasing the foot with the other hand. At the optimum moment in virtually full dorsiflexion, the thrust is applied with the tibial hand.

Tibio-taloid joint thrust (4)

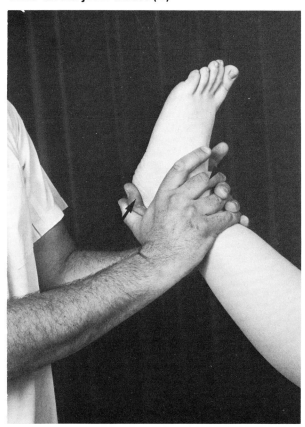

This hold for driving the tibia back on the talus is useful for small patients or children. It requires strong thumbs and a careful control of the tension sense to make it effective.

Tibio-taloid joint thrust (5)

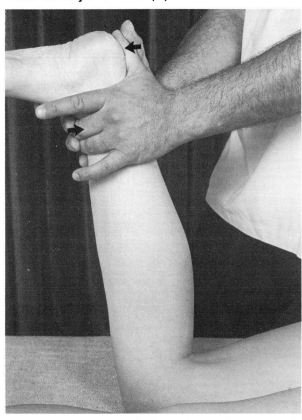

The hold shown here is similar to the previous one, only the patient is prone rather than supine. The degree of dorsiflexion is easily controlled in this hold by greater and lesser flexion of the knee.

Tibio-taloid joint thrust (6)

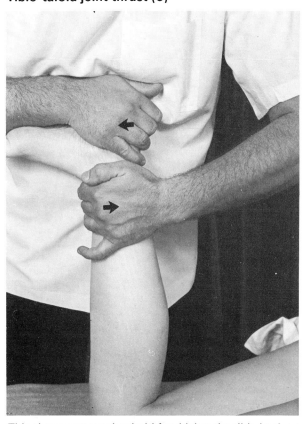

This shows yet another hold for driving the tibia back on the talus. Dorsiflexion is maintained by resting on the sole of the foot. All these holds can be altered to the opposite, to drive the talus and foot backwards on the tibia although this is rarely necessary in practice.

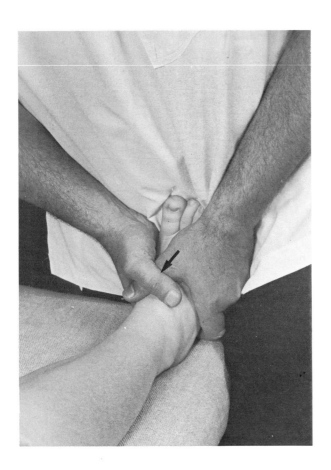

Figure of eight technique (1)

This and the next two pictures are part of a sequence which uses a so-called figure of eight procedure. The foot is buckled against the operator's abdomen and the thumbs are crossed. The operator firmly drives a force down one thumb, then while maintaining the buckling force, he directs the force across between the points of both thumbs. He then, while still maintaining the downward force, abducts, or adducts the foot, as the case may be and repeats the move in the other quadrants. The figure of eight has as its centre the crossed thumbs and the round ends of the eight are in fact flattened off.

Figure of eight technique (2)

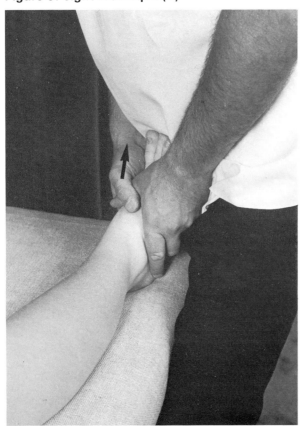

Figure of eight technique (3)

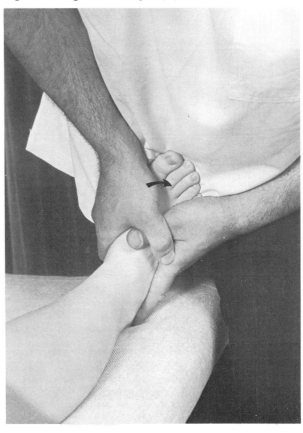

Figure of eight technique (4)

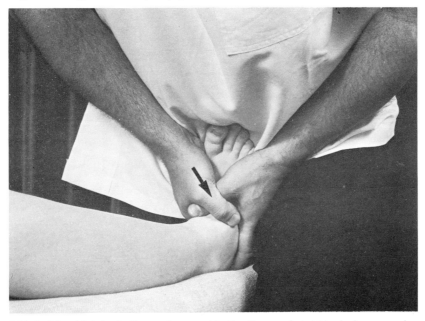

This hold, which is similar to that used in the figure of eight technique, can be used to drive individual bones in a specific direction. The foot is being buckled and the operator is keeping a firm pressure with the crossed thumbs and directing the thrust in at the middle cuneiform in this case.

Medial border of foot articulation and thrust (1)

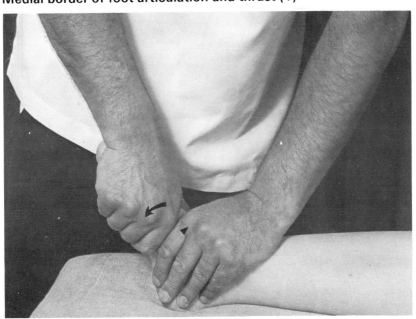

The medial border of the foot can be accessed in this hold. This picture shows the force being applied to the talo-navicular joint. The operator's left hand is holding back under the sustentaculum tali and the right hand is everting, plantar flexing and abducting the foot while maintaining a buckling force. The thrust is an emphasis of all these movements, particularly plantarflexion locally of the forefoot.

189

Medial border of foot articulation and thrust (2)

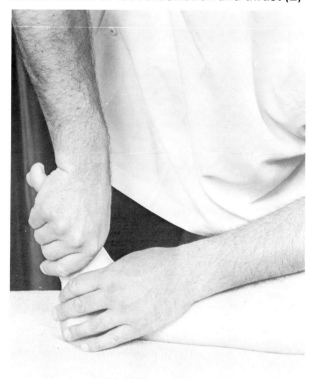

In this hold the operator is directing the force to the naviculo-cuneiform joint. The left hand is holding back on the navicular and the right is applying plantarflexion, eversion, abduction and compression. Note that the thrusting hand is nearly vertical to emphasise the compression element in the technique which minimises the other leverages.

Medial border of foot articulation and thrust (4)

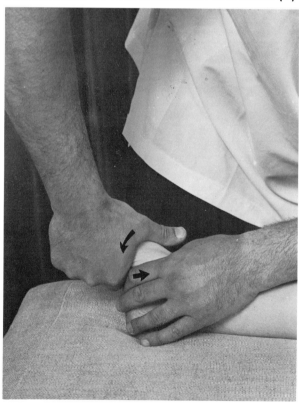

This shows the final position after the thrust to the navicular to medial cuneiform junction. Note that the foot has been pushed firmly into the table, the thrusting hand has descended and gone into relatively more palmar flexion than the previous picture, and that the operator's left hand has pulled firmly upwards on the navicular while stabilising the tibia.

Medial border of foot articulation and thrust (3)

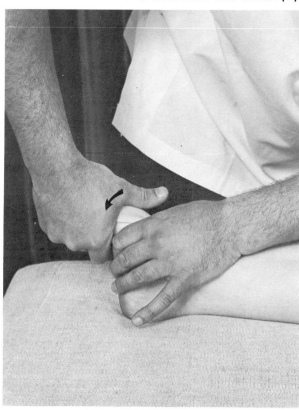

The thrust, or articulatory force is being directed here to the joint between the navicular and the medial cuneiform. This photo shows the mid thrust position. Note that the thrusting hand has everted the forefoot as well as abducting slightly and buckling the foot to utilise compression. Note also that the operator's left hand is holding the tibia to stabilise it.

Medial border of foot articulation and thrust (5)

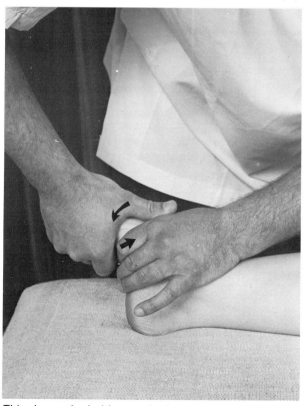

This shows the hold to apply the same principles as the last technique shown, only this time the target is the cuneiform to first metatarsal junction.

Medial border of foot articulation and thrust prone (1)

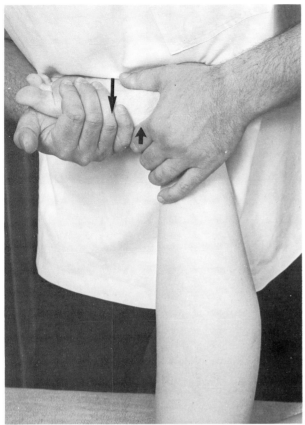

In the prone position the medial border of the foot is accessible using this hold. In this case the operator is articulating or thrusting the cuneiform towards the table while holding back on the navicular. Note that the operator is resting his abdomen on the lateral border of the foot to stabilise the technique. Note also that the operator is holding his own right forearm close into his side to increase the effect of body movement on the technique.

Medial border of foot articulation and thrust prone (2)

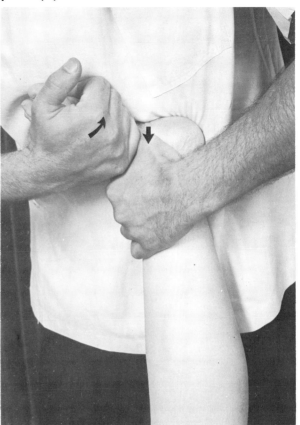

This hold is similar to the last one shown except that the operator is holding back on the cuneiform, in this case with the left hand, and is thrusting the first metatarsal bone into plantarflexion. Note that in this case the operator is holding his right forearm away from his side to increase the effect of the lever attempting to thrust up towards his own chest.

Inter-metatarsal mobilising (1)

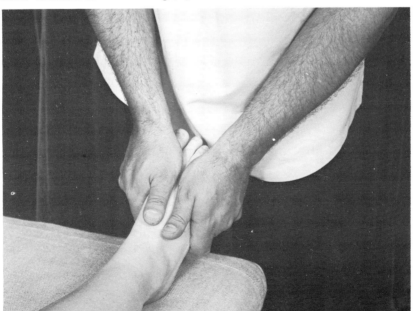

This hold is shown as a basic position to apply a shearing force to the midfoot in such a way as to reach all the mid tarsal joints. The hands can then be moved in a variety of directions while maintaining this basic hold to direct force where required.

Inter-metatarsal mobilising (2)

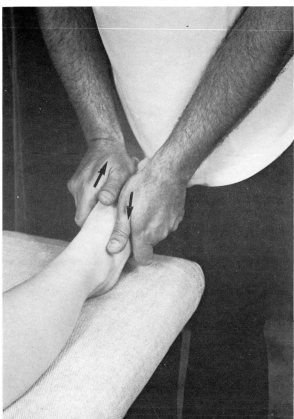

In this picture the operator has pushed his right hand into radial flexion and his left into ulnar flexion. This acts as a very powerful mobilising force on the midfoot when combined with the opposite movement. Note once again that the operator's arms are held well into his sides so that the body movement can perform the technique rather than just the hands.

Inter-metatarsal mobilising (3)

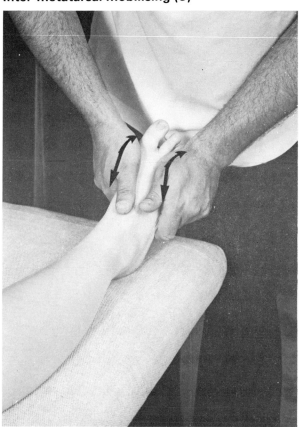

The arrows here should help to show the directions of force being used in this technique. They combine the general hold with the usual directions necessary.

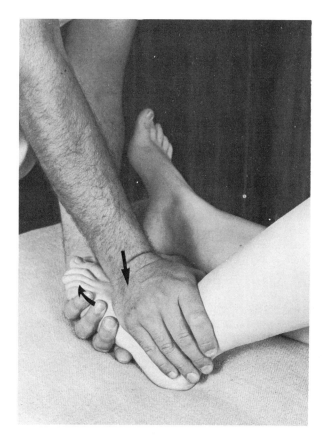

Middle cuneiform thrust

This hold can be used to direct a thrusting force at the middle cuneiform to mobilise it between the lateral and medial ones. The foot is being held into dorsiflexion by the opposite forces of the operator pulling the forefoot towards the ceiling and the midfoot towards the table specifically at the middle cuneiform by the application of the hypothenar eminence to it. By the use of compression, only very small amounts of inversion and eversion, and abduction and adduction are necessary to localise the force where required. This technique is not effective unless the preliminary slack is taken out with compression.

Thrust directed to individual tarsal bones

Articulation to sub-taloid joint

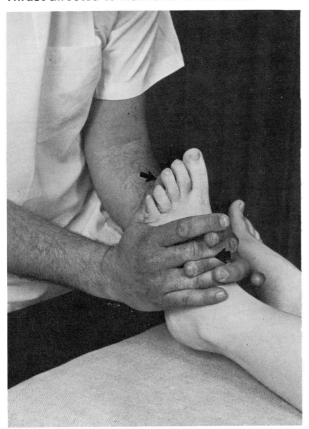

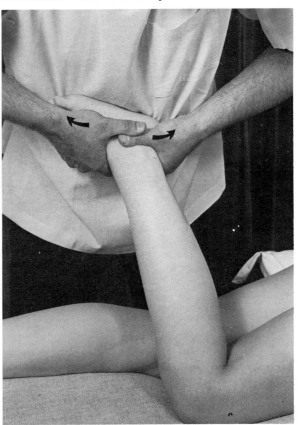

This hold can also be used to mobilise individual bones in the foot. It is being shown here as applied to the middle cuneiform. The slack is taken out and then the foot is abducted and adducted, as well as being inverted and everted until the force is accurately focused where the arrow is placed. Note the arms held close into the sides, and the thumbs maintaining dorsiflexion.

This hold is useful for mobilising the sub-taloid joint. The operator is maintaining firm contact with the sole of the foot and is then everting the foot by leaning over it and then rocking from side to side. This effectively reaches the sub-taloid joint on the medial border of the foot. The technique can also be performed by the operator holding a specific degree of dorsiflexion and then rocking into greater and lesser degrees of eversion.

Gapping thrust to sub-taloid joint

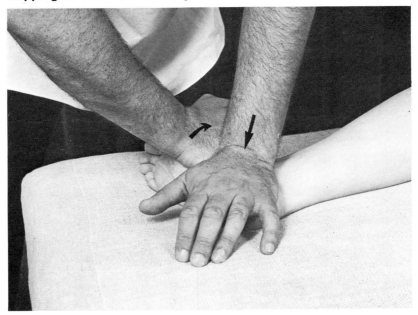

This hold allows a very specific force to be applied to the sub-taloid joint on the medial border of the foot. The operator places the foot on the table on its lateral border and then by a combination of forces focuses on the sub-taloid joint. The operator's right hand is inverting the navicular, and the left is pressing down on the posterior part of the calcaneum. By subtle changes in direction, once a compression force has been introduced, the sub-taloid becomes accessible.

Mobilising lateral border of foot

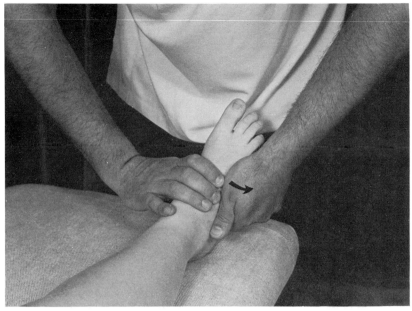

This hold is useful for mobilising the lateral border of the foot. The operator's right hand is gripping the lateral cuneiform, while the left is gripping the lateral two metatarsal bones and shearing them with the cuboid from the rest of the foot.

Cuboid thrust (1)

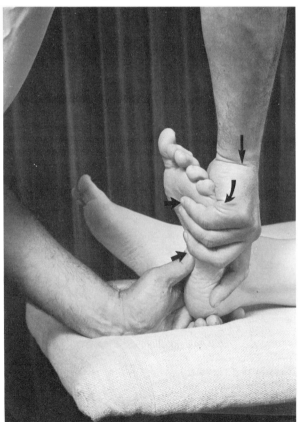

This shows one very effective hold for specifically mobilising or thrusting the cuboid. The foot is first dorsiflexed as shown to bring the medial border of the cuboid into prominence. The operator then takes a firm hold on it with his left thumb. The right hand then applies compression, plantar flexion and inversion with slight adduction to allow the thrust of the left thumb to drive the cuboid up. These two movements must of course be coincident.

Cuboid thrust (2)

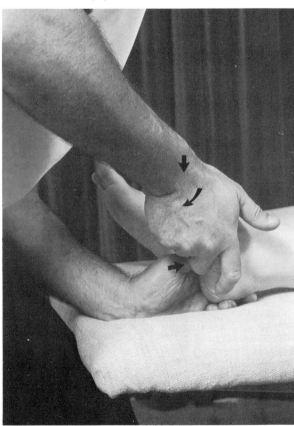

The final position of the hold used in the previous picture is shown here. The left thumb has thrust on the medial border of the cuboid, the right hand has inverted, plantar-flexed and adducted the lateral border of the foot.

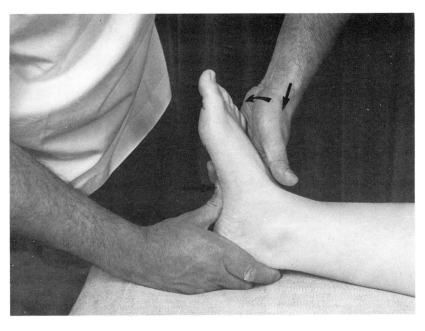

Cuboid thrust (3)

The previously shown cuboid technique is shown again here on the other foot for clarity.

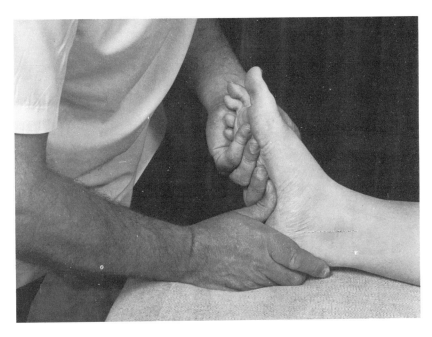

Cuboid thrust (4)

This shows the final position of the cuboid technique. For some operators' thumbs, this technique is impossible and then the thenar or hypothenar eminence can be substituted for the thrust.

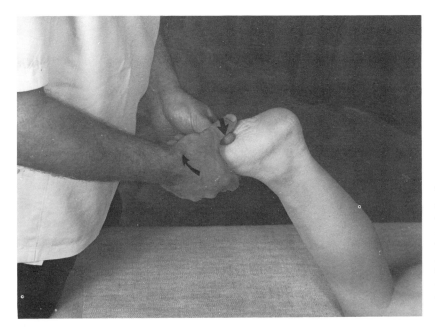

Prone cuboid thrust (1)

The prone position can be used for directing forces at most of the bones in the midfoot. In this particular case the operator has crossed his thumbs over the middle cuneiform and is inverting and adducting the foot and then driving the cuneiform towards the table with a flicking action. Note that to minimise force, it is important in this hold not to let the foot drop into plantarflexion.

195

Prone cuboid thrust (2)

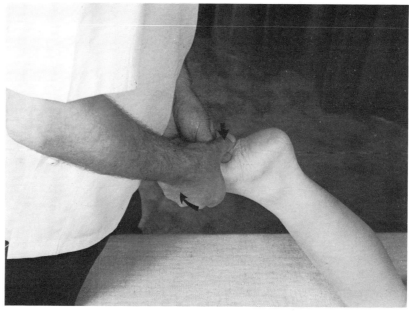

This picture shows the previous hold having been completed. Note that the thumbs have been pressed firmly into the sole of the foot, and that the operator's right hand has moved into more ulnar deviation than in the last picture.

Prone cuboid thrust (1)

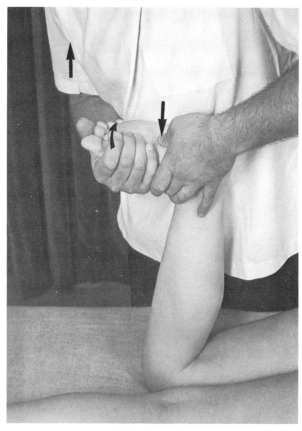

In this prone hold the operator has applied the left thumb to the medial border of the cuboid, and the right thenar eminence to the superior and lateral border of the foot. The right arm is held close to the side and the operator can then maintain dorsiflexion with the right fingers and inversion by shrugging the right shoulder. The left thumb can then thrust towards the table on the medial border of the cuboid.

Prone cuboid thrust (2)

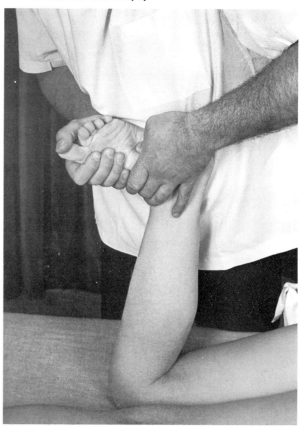

This shows the final position for the prone thrust to the medial border of cuboid. Once again the thenar or hypothenar eminence can be substituted for the thumb if necessary.

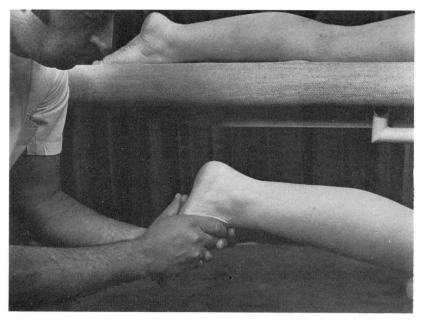

Cuboid thrust, leg over side (1)

This somewhat precarious hold can be used for mobilising the lateral border of the foot, particularly the cuboid. The operator has clasped the foot in such a way that the thumbs are crossed under the medial border of the cuboid, and the fingers are overlaying each other on the dorsum of the foot. The right hand is able to extend and thereby invert the foot, while the thenar eminence can maintain dorsiflexion by keeping a firm pressure on the sole.

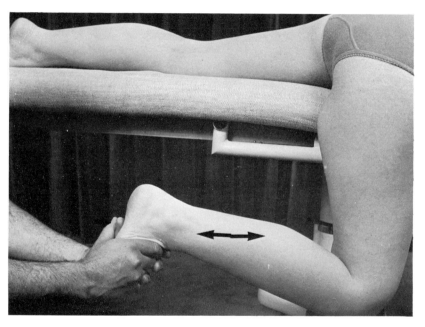

Cuboid thrust, leg over side (2)

This shows the oscillatory nature of the technique. The tibia is maintained virtually horizontal while the foot is pushed away and towards the operator maintaining the dorsiflexion.

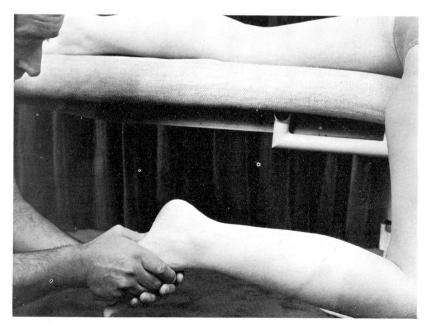

Cuboid thrust, leg over side (3)

The final position of the technique is shown here. Note that the foot is still substantially held in dorsiflexion, even though the thumbs have been thrust into the cuboid. The leg has been moved back and forth and on one of the backward movements towards the operator, the thumbs are used to stop the cuboid, even though the leg carries on. If this thrust is performed in plantar-flexion, a great deal more force is necessary.

197

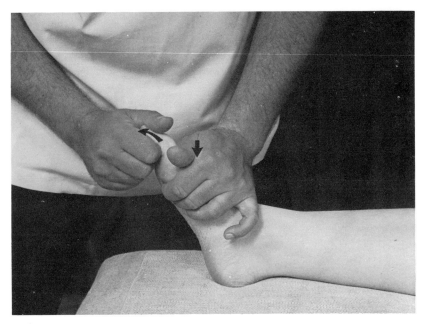

Inter-phalangeal gapping

The hold shown here is effective for gapping the interphalangeal joint of the first toe. The left hand is holding back on the first metatarsal and first phalange. The right hand is inducting traction and plantarflexion.

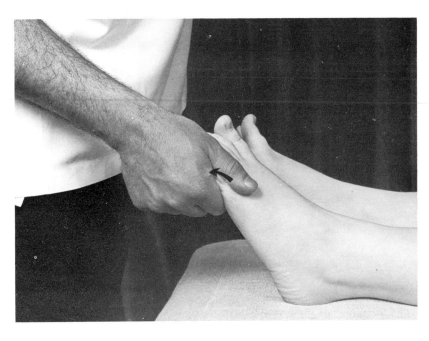

Metatarso-phalangeal joint gapping (1)

The metatarso-phalangeal joints can be mobilised using this hold. Traction, a small degree of abduction or adduction, a small degree of circumduction in either direction to optimise the tension, and then plantarflexion are induced.

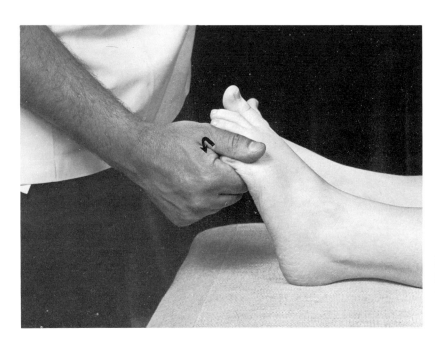

Metatarso-phalangeal joint gapping (2)

This shows the completion of the technique for separating the metatarso-phalangeal joints.

198

Section L
Miscellaneous techniques

Mobilising hyoid

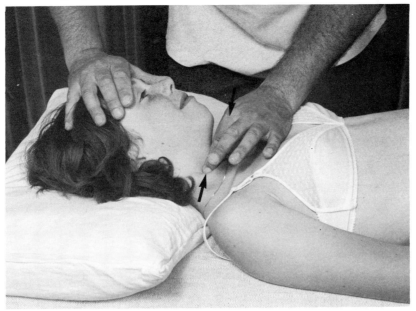

One hold used for mobilising the hyoid bone is shown here. The cornua are gently clasped between the finger and thumb and then the hyoid is carefully moved from side to side, or up and down as deemed necessary. If stronger mobilising is considered necessary, the operator can hold down on the hyoid as the patient is asked to swallow. This can be even further strengthened if the patient's head is turned away from the side being mobilised.

Stretching masseter

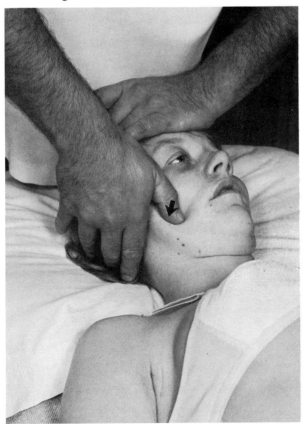

When working on the temporo-mandibular joint the operator can use this hold to perform a strong graduated stretch on the masseter to allow freer movement of the joint. Note that the operator has stabilised the patient's head with the other hand.

Mobilising tempero-mandibular joint

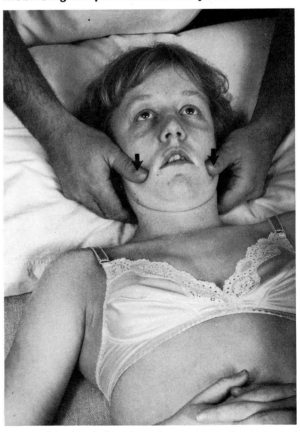

This double-handed hold can be used to perform bilateral stretch to the temporo-mandibular joint. The patient must be asked to co-operate by letting the jaw sag.

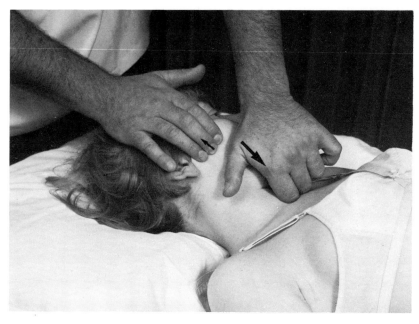

Stretching tempero-mandibular joint

The hold shown here is useful to stretch one temporo-mandibular joint by holding back on the maxilla, and carefully prising the mandible away from it.

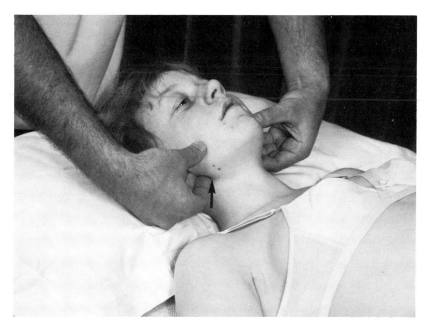

Antero-posterior articulation

If antero-posterior movement is considered necessary, this hold can be used. The angle of the mandible is often very sensitive, and care must be taken to avoid inducing discomfort in this hold which will reduce its effectiveness due to tension in the patient.

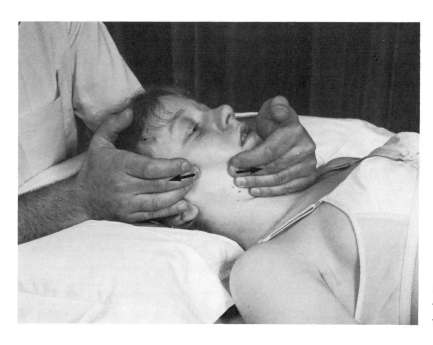

Unilateral stretching

This hold is useful to stretch the tempero-mandibular joint unilaterally.

Tempero-mandibular joint stretching over fulcrum

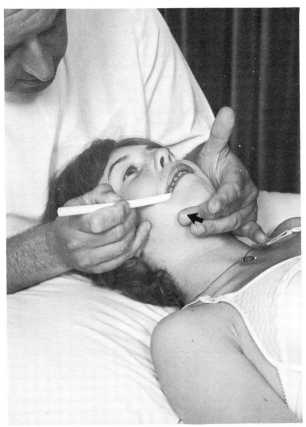

If a fulcrum is introduced into the mouth between the back teeth, pressure upwards on the point of the jaw will tend to prise the joint apart on the side of the fulcrum. Different thicknesses of fulcrum will affect different quadrants of the joint.

Lymphatic pump

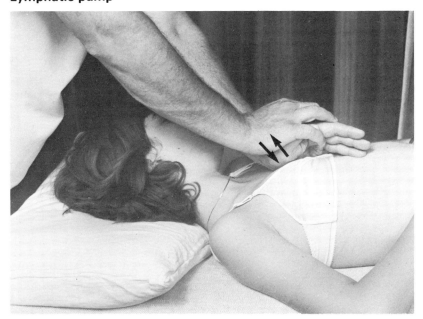

This hold forms the starting point for the "Lymphatic Pump". This technique consists of a rapidly oscillating to-and-fro pressure and release on the sternum. This must be co-incident with exhalation by the patient. The purpose is to "pump" the static lymph from the cysterna chyli into the general circulatory system, and thereby aid auto-immune responses. Whether this effect is in fact achieved is open to discussion, however the technique is an ancient osteopathic classic.

Vibration to sinus

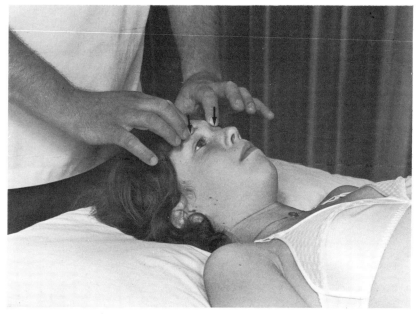

The hold shown here is sometimes used to apply vibration to the supra-orbital nerve to assist in promoting drainage in a case of sinusitis. Alternatively rotatory friction can be applied to this site for the same purpose.

Vibration to sinus

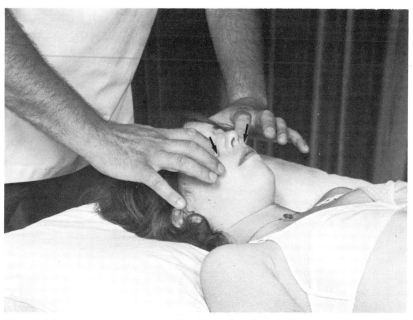

The position shown here is to apply either vibration or rotatory pressure to the maxillary nerve emission point. This is designed to assist in aiding drainage in a case of sinusitis.

INDEX